Katahdin or Bust

Increasing Your Odds of Enjoying Hiking and Backpacking

By

Gail Hinshaw

April 10, 2018

KATAHDIN OR BUST: INCREASING YOUR ODDS OF
ENJOYING HIKING AND BACKPACKING

Copyright © 2018 Gail L. Hinshaw

Printed in the United States

ISBN-978-1-7321643-0-7

Cover and interior formatting by Sweet 'N Spicy Designs

Final Edit by Jim Hawkins

All photographs by the Author unless otherwise noted

Cover photograph by Jennifer Kee

Printed by Hinshaw and Associates, Inc.
789 Seven Pines Drive
Saddlebrooke, Missouri 65630

Visit www.KatahdinOrBust.com

Dedication

This book is dedicated to two individuals: Sheila Hinshaw, my wife of close to fifty years, for supporting me in hiking the Appalachian Trail and Peter Conti, also known by his trail name as Flash 52, who serves as an inspiration to me every day.

It takes a special woman to become an *Appalachian Trail Widow* for several months while her husband treks through the woods. I thank my wife for looking the other way as expensive equipment showed up on our doorstep as I worked to get the right gear I thought I needed. Without complaint, she held down our home and did double duty to cover the tasks I would have performed if I had been home. Her generous spirit gave me the most precious gift of all—time to pursue my passion.

I met Flash 52 on the trail in Pennsylvania in 2016. Flash has such a great motivational story to tell; he deserves more than just a mention in a dedication. Therefore, I have put a special section in the Appendix, sharing a part of his story that will serve as a motivator for anybody wanting to hike the Appalachian Trail, commonly referred to as the AT. Be sure to read how he hiked the AT to heal the constant pain in his leg due to a motorcycle accident. I kept saying to myself, "If Flash 52 could do this, so can I!" Hopefully, others will say the same thing after reading his story.

Acknowledgments

Writing any book is practically impossible without the aid of others. Books of this nature also need more sources of information to cover a topic properly.

The list of people I need to acknowledge in writing this book starts with my wife, Sheila. In addition to allowing me the time away to hike the AT and supporting me along the way, she also spent hours proofreading this book, making corrections, and offering suggestions to make it better.

Special acknowledgment needs to go to Dana and Jennifer Kee (Trail names Atlas and Matchmaker) who not only became great friends but aided in working out the details and nuances of using the "Self Double-Shuttle." It was their willingness to put their trust in a crazy old man who proposed an unorthodox way of hiking the AT that eventually will lead more people than ever before not just to hike the AT, but to enjoy it as well.

My wife and I are fortunate to have bestselling author, Cara Bristol, and her husband, DH, as next-door neighbors. It was Cara's willingness to share her knowledge of writing and publishing that was so helpful in bringing this book to fruition.

I must also recognize a dear friend, Jim Hawkins, who supplied his in-depth knowledge of the English language to keep me from looking like a complete fool. It was his final editing that makes me look like an author.

Finally, I want to thank Dr. Warren Doyle for his insightful Foreword. It is a wonderful feeling when the person who has hiked more miles on the Appalachian Trail than anyone else agrees with your thoughts about how to enjoy the trail.

Gail Hinshaw

Contents

Foreword

This book is a most welcome addition to the literature of the Appalachian Trail. It is an easy-to-read narrative on how to increase the chances of realizing one's dream of walking the entire Appalachian Trail either in one continuous stretch of time (i.e. thru-hiking) of over a number of years (i.e. section-hiking).

For over 45 years, there has been an abysmal failure rate on people attempting to walk the entire AT (i.e. 75-80%). What a tremendous waste of time and money, not to mention the negativity of thousands of dreams not realized. AT hopefuls continue to make the same simple mistakes year after year.

THIS DOES NOT HAVE TO HAPPEN! I have spent almost 45 years as a grassroots, committed AT trail educator proving this. Yes, it is better to be a SMART hiker than a STRONG hiker. Yes, it is better to focus more on THOUGHTS/FEELINGS rather than on THINGS (i.e. equipment).

Mr. Hinshaw's book focuses on the more relevant areas of AT preparation. His emphasis on day-hiking the trail is long overdue and especially relevant to hikers over the age of forty. He points out the common sense obvious that older hikers have more discretionary time and money to afford day-hiking the trail (which doesn't have to be expensive). Carrying 5-10 lbs. as a day-hiker is easier on the body than carrying 25-40 lbs. as a backpacker, especially for older hikers who injure more easily and take longer to heal.

It is my hope, as well as the author's, that this book will help future hiker hopefuls realize their AT dreams. However, do not try a hike of the entire AT without at least a 10-day backpack/or continuous day hike under your feet. Some experience hiking in northern New England offers a more realistic picture than hiking in the southeast and the midwest. The only way that hiking the entire trail can be fun or enjoyable is accepting the fact that walking the entire trail is inherently slow, difficult. and uncomfortable. Or as AT hiker trail named Model T has said, "Walking on the happy side of misery."

So, enjoy the book. Get out there day-hiking with smarts rather than brute strength. And, don't let anyone say you are not an AT hiker if you don't carry a backpack. Just tell them that you thought that was what mules were for.

Warren Doyle
37,000-miler
Founder: ALDHA(honorary life member)
Founder/Director: Appalachian Trail Institute at the Appalachian Folk School
ATC Life Member
www.warrendoyle.com

Preface

The Appalachian Trail. Just the name sparks a desire to discover this wonderful treasure that travels 2,200 miles between Georgia and Maine.

My Appalachian Trail journey, and ultimately the desire to write this book, started a few months before retirement. My wife of 45 years understood it was now time for me to do some of the things I had delayed because of supporting our family. One of those items was to go hiking and backpacking, an activity I learned to love as a youth when I worked as a Ranger at Philmont Scout Ranch in Cimarron, New Mexico.

My first thought about doing something special was to hike across the Grand Canyon. I started researching the equipment needed and the logistics required to fulfill this trip. Several months later, I flew a third of the way across the country to Las Vegas, rented a car, and drove five hours to the canyon. I then took a four-hour shuttle from the south rim to the north rim, spent one night in a campground on the north rim, and then hiked for six days back to my rental car on the south side of the canyon. I wanted to spend as much time in the canyon as the park service would allow. There was no way I would go to all that trouble and expense to simply blow by what I came to experience.

After hiking the canyon, I started looking for another challenge. I realized a short section hike on the AT as it is commonly called, would easily fit my travel plans and schedule. I was going to Washington, D.C. anyway, so why not go a week early and hike a part of the AT? I could take a train to Harpers Ferry, WV, from Washington, DC, shuttle ride 40 miles up the trail, hike across Maryland back to Harpers Ferry, then finish with a train ride back to Washington DC. Plus, I would stay the first and last night at the Teahorse Hostel, giving me the opportunity to get a feel for the atmosphere and culture of the trail. I already had my equipment from hiking the Grand Canyon, so why not?

Once I completed this trip, the Appalachian Trail bug bit me. Plus, I had earned the trail name Dr. Fix-it, given to me by fellow AT hiker Ohio Grass Man. Trail names are used by most of the folks on the AT for several reasons, one of which is to keep everyone anonymous. They also give a starting point for conversation, explaining how you got your trail name because these names reflect something about the person or an event that had happened involving the person. What is the basis for my trail name? I was fixing equipment for people.

Now that I had this AT affliction, driven partly by having a trail name that obligated me to fix things for people along the AT, I started planning my hike. This time, however, I committed much more effort to research and planning and more money for equipment. After all, the hike would take six months, not simply six days. Instead of carrying my equipment 40 miles, it would be over 2,000. Naturally, my decision-making process turned away from trying to save a few bucks to try to save a few pounds, and then later to shave a few ounces. My planning got more intense and testing my equipment got much more serious until at last, I had my plan completed with the backpacking gear I felt was great. I figured both my plans and my gear would probably change along the way as I gained experience and knowledge.

At last, the day arrived to head out on an epic journey of a lifetime. I had researched the best time and place to start hiking, (first of May and in the middle of the trail but this will all be explained later), so off to the airport and on to Washington, DC Reagan International Airport. A subway ride plus an Amtrak train ride later, I was standing outside the train station in Harpers Ferry, West Virginia with another gentleman and a married couple I had met on the train. They were planning to hike the AT as well. Hikers are easy to spot with their backpacks. During my short section hike the previous year, I discovered smell could also be used to determine who the hikers were who had been on the trail for a while.

It had been a long day, and I was ready to find a place to sleep that first night away from home. Because we all had different plans, our small group of hikers split up but knew we would meet up later on the trail. I headed to the Teahorse Hostel which I had used the year prior. It was such a wonderful place; I had to return.

The next morning after a waffle breakfast, I headed north. My plan for the starting day was to only hike about six miles to the first hikers' shelter north of Harpers Ferry. With over 260 of the shelters spaced across the entire length of the AT, you can plan to find one every seven to ten miles. Most shelters provide space for six to ten hikers to sleep as well as having a source of water in the area. A campsite for tents as well as a privy were almost always close to the shelters.

From my prior year's section hike, I had the opportunity to meet a few thru-hikers or hikers that were planning to hike the entire trail within a year's time. I noticed that most of these hikers were young, in great shape, and obsessed with how many miles they had hiked that day. There were a few older or senior hikers as I call them, doing short sections of the trail. Occasionally I had met an older hiker who was a thru-hiker, but not as many as I would have expected.

"Everybody tells me how far they hiked, but nobody tells me what they saw."

Louis Amore

After a few hours of hiking, I arrived at the shelter and claimed a spot inside on the shelter floor for my air mattress and sleeping quilt. Before long, other hikers started showing up. The first to arrive were those who had just started their hike at Harpers Ferry including the couple I had met on the train. Later that night they would get the trail names of On Hold and Time Out as they had put their lives *on hold* and were taking *time out* of their careers to hike the AT. They were planning to hike the north half of the trail first then returning to Harpers Ferry and heading south to complete their thru-hike. A hike of this style is called a "flip-flop" which is what I intended to do as well. As the evening wore on, thru-hikers started to arrive. It appeared the major item of conversation among the thru-hikers was how many miles they did that day. That evening, all I could think about was a quote from Louis Amore, the great western historical fiction writer, who said, "Everybody tells me how far they hiked, but nobody tells me what they saw."

As the sun set, and after everybody had eaten their dinner, I learned it was now hiker midnight and time for all to crawl into bed.

The next morning, I was off for a 57-day hike that would take me to Dalton, Massachusetts, a fourth of the entire AT. Somewhere in Pennsylvania, I started traveling with a gentleman with the trail name of Flash 52. He was traversing the AT to heal a nerve damaged leg. I mention him here because there was one thing that made him different than the other hikers, something that would lead me to rethink how to hike the AT. He had a car. He used his car to carry the medical equipment he needed to stretch and exercise his leg. He also used the car to transport other items used on the trail as well. He would drive his car up the trail a distance equal to one to five days of hiking, get someone to shuttle him back to where he had left off the trail, and then hike to his car. When he got to the car, he had wheels to drive to town and not only resupply but maybe stay in a hotel to exercise his leg in the hotel swimming pool, get a great meal, see a movie, and a ton of other options. Being able to change one's camping gear every few days was an obvious benefit over those hikers who had to call home to get other gear. It was also fantastic to be able to buy food in bulk and store the excess until needed.

It was during this time I began to think of added ways to make hiking the AT more enjoyable. I noticed how young hikers would bound over rocks as they moved down the trail while I was slowly, carefully, taking one step at a time, trying not to hurt myself. I soon realized there were several differences between older hikers like myself and the youngsters on the trail. I started to interview older or senior hikers for advice about hiking the AT as well as talking to other hikers on alternatives to the brutal thru-hiking mentality. Before long, I realized I was amassing a large body of knowledge about how to make hiking the AT doable as well as more enjoyable for more people. It was from this knowledge that I began to think about writing a book.

I was forced off the trail at Dalton, Massachusetts after I developed "exercise-induced peroneal neuropathy" in my feet and hands, or as a doctor so kindly put it, "You hiked so much you screwed up your feet and hands!"

By the time I got home, my wife and I had decided I should continue my hike when I was physically able to do so. During my convalescence, I had breakfast with some of my retired friends. Many of them had been following my hike via Facebook, so naturally, they had dozens of questions. As I answered their questions, it became obvious many would like to do what I was doing but felt they physically were not able to hike the Appalachian Trail. I told them about how Flash 52 had a car and that I was planning to buy a used minivan and outfit it with my camping gear, food, a mattress, and anything else that might be useful on the trail. Once this idea was explained, the conversation began to change from "can't" to "maybe." It was during this time that one neighbor, considerably older than I, had been sitting quietly for this entire time, asked two simple questions. First, he asked: "Gail, I know you will not be able to finish the entire trail this year, so are you going back next year to complete it?" When I affirmed that was my plan, he then said with tears in his eyes, "I've always wanted to hike the AT but did not think I would ever be able to do it. With what you said, I think I could hike at least part of it. Would you mind if I came out to the trail next year and hiked a few days with you?"

What could I say but yes? I would be honored to do whatever I could to make sure he had a wonderful experience on the trail. And with that, this book was born for not only for my senior friends but for the thousands of people who do not necessarily want to backpack the AT but want to enjoy it in some fashion or another.

Introduction

It had been four days since I had a shower. I stunk so bad the flies started leaving me alone. My muscles hurt in places I did not know I had places. As I continued putting one foot in front of the other, pushing my body over yet another boulder in the middle of the trail, I started to cry. I thought, "Man, how can I be so blessed? I'm pushing 70 and hiking the Appalachian Trail!"

There are a ton of books telling how to hike the AT, but very few, if any, on how to enjoy it.

And so starts the reason for this book. I want other people to experience the joy of the Appalachian Trail. Hiking the AT is a daunting task, but because of my experience as an old geezer hiking the trail, I discovered there are many of ways to enjoy the Appalachian Trail without all the pain. The information and hiking strategies outlined in this book can help anyone hike and relish their experience. There are a ton of books telling how to hike the AT, but very few, if any, on how to enjoy it. There is a significant difference. My experience tells me that many of the people who hike the entire AT in one year end up feeling like an employee of the trail with a job that needs to be done every day with quarterly reviews always coming up. They lose the joy of their hike. This book explains how to avoid losing that joy and instead, become a boss of their hike and start loving the AT experience.

In 2017, approximately 4,000 people studied, planned, bought $1,500 to $4,000 of equipment, set aside four to seven months of their lives, budgeted $4,000 to $7,000 to spend while hiking, and arranged to get to a trailhead. These activities were all done with the anticipation of thru-hiking the Appalachian Trail. However, 80% of these people would eventually fail! Many of these hikers lost their joy of the trail;

others ran out of money, some got physically got hurt. No matter what the reason, a process that has an 80% failure rate is the wrong process!

To put an 80% failure rate into perspective, this is like dropping eight out of every ten babies you pick up, or out of every ten airplanes that take off, eight will crash! People have had to accept this same high failure rate of the current AT hiking process, until NOW!

This book explains an entirely new, innovative approach to long distance hiking. Originally conceived to allow more seniors to enjoy hiking and backpacking, it is becoming a game changer for those people who are in the 80% failure group. For many, mainly that 20 % who have been successful with their thru-hikes, this book is highly controversial. However, when one remembers that everybody needs to simply hike their own hike, then, perhaps, this book is exactly what 80% of the Appalachian Trail hikers need.

While this book has dozens of tips and hacks to make hiking more enjoyable as well as information to aid in the planning of an AT hike, it is by no means complete unto itself. This book's content comes from several places in addition to my personal experience from hiking over 3,000 miles, including close to 2,000 miles of the AT. The reference section in the Appendix gives several added sources of information that are invaluable in planning an AT hike.

Another source of information came from interviews with 125 senior hikers I met while hiking the AT. Among this group of senior hikers was Dale Sanders, trail name of Grey Beard. On October 26th, 2017, Dale made history in becoming the oldest person at age 82, to hike the entire Appalachian Trail in one calendar year! It was from Dale and the other seniors I interviewed that I created the ten points of wisdom for the chapter titled *Advice from the Trail*.

The final base of information for this book comes from researching a variety of sources, both printed and Internet-based. Most of this information was verified either personally or through secondary sources. However, I am no expert. People thinking of hiking the AT need to do their own study and hopefully, this book will be a great starting point for their research.

Because I am a senior citizen, I was intrigued by discovering four major differences between senior hikers and younger hikers. While these observations will not be true all the time, they are more times than not.

1. Senior hikers have more discretionary time

Younger hikers have a definite time to do their hiking. They are limited by school or need to get back to work. Seniors, on the other hand, are generally retired and are fulfilling a lifelong bucket list item. Therefore, if their hike takes eight months or eight years, it is about fulfilling a dream without the pressure of other obligations.

2. Senior hikers have more discretionary money

Younger hikers have a limited or fixed budget for their hike. Many told me they had to complete their hike before their money ran out so the more expenses they can avoid the longer they would get to hike and hopefully complete the trail. Seniors, on the other hand, have a retirement income so all they need to do is keep living and their money will keep coming every month. This recurring money source also gives them the ability to buy lightweight gear as well as change out and replace gear as appropriate.

3. Seniors injure more easily

I watched in amazement as younger hikers jumped up and then down from boulders along the trail. Being an older hiker, my body never hesitates to inform me when I play idiot and jar something out of place. If I hiked like the younger folks, I would have to hire a chiropractor to hike with me, so I could get put back into place every time I made such a move. I saw younger hikers cover 18 to 30 miles a day and appear not to suffer the next day. I could hike ten to fourteen miles a day and be fine, but when I pushed for more miles than that, my body told me I had made a stupid decision.

4. Seniors take longer to heal from injuries

I have had four major physical problems while hiking the AT, all of which involved my lower legs. The first was *exercise-induced peripheral neuropathy* in my hands and feet which the doctor said could take up to one year to heal. The second injury I thought was a stress fracture but turned out to simply be *severe tendonitis* in my right foot. The third major physical problem I experienced on the AT was *shin splints* in my left leg which took four weeks to heal, and finally, the last medical problem I had was *plantar fasciitis* in my left foot. I had seen younger hikers with similar ailments take a couple of days to a couple of weeks off the trail then continue their journey. My periods of convalescence were from four to ten weeks.

It is these differences that make most of the suggestions in this book for enjoying the Appalachian Trail especially proper for seniors. However, younger hikers will find many of the suggestions worth their consideration. If nothing else, perhaps young hikers can send a copy of this book to their parents, so they can better understand why their child is out hiking in the woods for six months. Then maybe, their parents will take the time to get out and enjoy the trail themselves.

In concluding this introduction, I want to share ten critical bits of information I learned through the course of my hike. Had I had known just this information when I started my AT quest, I feel I would have had a good chance of completing my thru-hike. These items are covered throughout the rest of this book, but I will summarize them here.

1. The less you carried, the better your body can hand the trail.
2. Listen to your body. Do not try to carry too much, too far, too soon.
3. Healthy lower legs and feet are critical to enjoying the trail.

4. Selecting the proper brand, type, and style of shoe along with a proper insole is critical to pain-free hiking.

5. Shoes can be laced a dozen diverse ways and selecting the proper lacing technique is also critical to pain-free hiking.

6. Hiking shoes will wear out from the inside and should be thrown out after 400 to 500 miles on the trail.

7. Muscle stretching is important.

8. Selecting the proper trekking pole can save nerve damage to the hands.

9. Never increase weekly mileage hiked by more than 10% from the previous week to keep your body from rebelling.

10. Proper nutrition is vital to have the energy to hike over the long haul.

> *"The AT is more than just a footpath. It is a community as well as an experience that changes lives."*
>
> **Dr. Fix-it**

Chapter 1
What is the Appalachian Trail?

The Appalachian Trail is a hiking trail that runs approximately 2,200 miles from the top of Springer Mountain in Georgia to the top of Mount Katahdin in Baxter State Park, Maine. It is the world's longest hiking-only trail. No bikes, vehicles, or pack animals are allowed, although dogs are welcome in most areas. It runs through fourteen different states, eight national forests, six national park units, and various state parks and forests. There are about 260 shelters; most have a water source, privy, and camping sites. One is never far from civilization as the trail crosses a road an average of every four miles. AND, according to Flash 52, "there is food on every road," it just depends on how far off your path you want to go to satisfy your hunger.

The entire trail is marked with white blazes or paint marks approximately 2" by 6". These blazes are painted on trees as well as on rocks, sidewalks, roads, posts, bridge abutments, utility poles, or anything else that is handy. They can vary in distance from being so close you can always see one in front of you, to times when they are hundreds of yards apart. Side trails are marked with the same size of painted blazes but in blue instead of white. These blue blazed trails can lead to just about any feature on the trail such as a spring, campsite, shelter, privy, parking lot, side road, or bad weather bypass trail, overlook, or anything else that might be of interest to hikers. Above the timberline, the trail may also be marked with human-made piles or stacks of rocks called cairns.

The trail goes through the following states. The miles through each state, as of the time of this writing, are shown to the right of each state.

Appalachian Trail States with Mileage

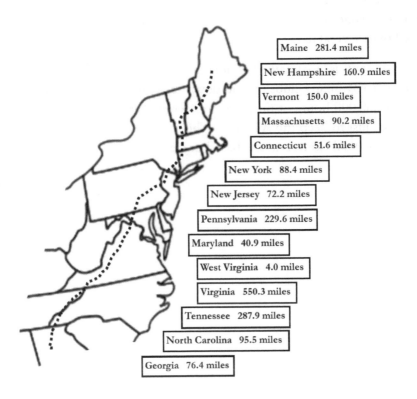

Maine   281.4 miles

New Hampshire   160.9 miles

Vermont   150.0 miles

Massachusetts   90.2 miles

Connecticut   51.6 miles

New York   88.4 miles

New Jersey   72.2 miles

Pennsylvania   229.6 miles

Maryland   40.9 miles

West Virginia   4.0 miles

Virginia   550.3 miles

Tennessee   287.9 miles

North Carolina   95.5 miles

Georgia   76.4 miles

Hiking the entire AT is no walk in the park. The good news is there are lots of people, churches, and even businesses that offer support, both physical and emotional, to those on the trail. Hikers receive help along the trail by an entire community of volunteers called *Trail Angels*; many are former hikers. Towns along the trail have organizations that go out of their way to support hikers. Churches open their doors and their purses to assist trekkers. Any type of help offered to hikers is referred to as *Trail Magic*. Trail magic can be things as simple as a ride to town or as complex as large meals, prepared for all hikers in the area and may be offered over several days.

The trail is maintained primarily by an army of volunteers belonging to 31 hiking clubs up and down the entire trail. It is estimated that over 250,000 hours of time is volunteered every year by over 6,000 volunteers, just to keep the AT open. The trail itself is managed by The Appalachian Trail Conservatory, based in Harpers Ferry, West Virginia.

> *"To appreciate the present, one must know the struggles of the past."*
>
> Jim Paisley, Historian and Educator

Chapter 2
The History of the Appalachian Trail

In 1921, an Irish American named Benton MacKaye, conceived the Appalachian trail. It was his vision that saw a walking trail along the backbone of the Appalachian Mountains, connecting various farms and wilderness work study farms. The initial trail was completed in 1937, 16 years after it was first proposed.

Benton MacKaye's vision included shelters that would allow people a place to stop, spend the night, and to enjoy the outdoors. Mr. MacKaye never envisioned people would hike the entire trail, especially in one long hike. Instead, he thought people would hike to a shelter, spend time there, then go to the top of a mountain, see the overlook, and then head back down. It is for this reason the AT goes across the top of mountains instead of simply going around them as many long-distance trails do.

While Mr. MacKaye first thought of the AT, it was an attorney, Myron Avery, who eventually would muster the forces to see the trail completed. As mentioned earlier, the trail is managed by Appalachian Trail Conservancy with 31 trail clubs each maintaining a portion. The US Forest Service, as well as the National Parks Service, each play an important part of managing and supporting portions as well. The trail is currently on some type of public land for approximately 99 plus percent of its length.

The actual trail is constantly changing due to various safety and environmental, as well as legal, issues along its length. Each year, the Appalachian Trail Conservancy readjusts the official length. What is important is that all users of the trail keep in mind what a privilege it is to have such an asset to enjoy and the best way to keep this asset available for generations to come is to follow the rules and do what they can to protect the trail. Every year a small minority of hikers do stupid things that cause the loss of privileges along the trail. For this reason, the remaining majority must go above and beyond the norm to be courteous and thankful to all the people they meet along the way.

For more information about the history, legends, and stories about the AT, J.R. "Model-T" Tate has written about the traditions and lore of the Appalachian Trail in his book, *Walkin' with the Ghost Whisperers.*

> ## *"If it was easy, everybody would be doing it".*
>
> **Dads of the World**

Chapter 3
Who Hikes the Appalachian Trail?

Currently, every year around 4,000 people attempt to hike the entire trail while three to four million people hike at least a part. Only one in five hikers that intend to hike the entire trail in a year will complete their hike. Most of these want-to-be thru-hikers fall into one of the following categories:

Recent college graduates

The first major group of hikers is those young people who have just graduated college and want to hike the AT before joining the real world. When I visited with people from this group of hikers, I learned some of their reasons for being on the trail. Many want to hike it before starting a professional career that would keep them from having the time, while others wish to create a resume item which proves their willingness to make sacrifices to carry out goals. Some stated that they wanted to do something they could look back on for encouragement when they got depressed or questioned their ability or worth.

Recently discharged military personnel

Earl Schafer, the first recognized AT thru-hiker, was a WWII veteran who said he hiked the trail to "walk the war out of his system." While recently discharged military personnel was a rather small group in comparison to the others, I felt compelled to include them here to encourage our country's veterans to consider hiking the AT to help them get through a tough time in their lives. I never hesitate to visit with veterans when they want to talk to me about the trail or anything else they want to discuss. It is the least we all can do for these people that we owe so much.

Middle-aged professionals

The third major group of hikers is those folks who have a career, have always wanted to hike the AT, but never found the time to do so. Many believe as they grow older, the door of ability to hike the trail may close. If this group of people is ever going to hike the AT, they feel the sooner, the better. Some middle-aged hikers have been given time off by their employers but have a fixed deadline to complete their venture. Others have found themselves unemployed and so have decided now is the opportunity. Whatever the reason, most have thought about hiking the AT for a long time.

Recent retirees

The fourth major group of AT hikers is recent retirees that have put off hiking the AT for many years but finally have the time to fulfill this dream. In addition to fulfilling a dream, some desire to leave a legacy for their family to remember what their grandparent accomplished. Of the four groups, recent retirees have the highest completion rate. When starting at the southern end of the AT and hiking north, my experience was there appeared not to be many older hikers among the mix. However, by the time I reached the north end of the trail, a high percentage of the hikers completing the trail were older people due to the high rate of loss of younger hikers.

Groups

The final group of people almost always plan to do short sections of the trail and not planning to thru-hike the AT. There were formal clubs, like scouts or church youth groups as well as informal groups of friends or family. In most of these situations, it was the journey and not the destination that drove their enjoyment of the trail.

> *"Things are more enjoyable if I know and understand the why."*
>
> **Matchmaker, 2017 AT Hiker**

Chapter 4

Why do People Hike the Appalachian Trail?

For each person who hikes the AT, there is a reason. Many hikers have more than one. My informal research did reveal, however, a correlation between the strength of a person's reason for hiking the trail and actual completion of the trail. I say this based on the time I was hiking at the north end of the trail and met a lot of hikers about to complete their thru-hike. When I asked *why*, their reasons were much more solid and sure than when I asked the same question at the start of the trail. Perhaps these answers became solid while on the trail and were not present at the beginning. Either way, people who complete their thru-hike seem to have a solid and compelling reason for having spent several months of their lives and several thousand dollars to hike the AT.

. . .the people who believe the American Dream is to own your own home, have never hiked the Appalachian Trail.

According to some, the people who believe the American Dream is to own your own home, have never hiked the Appalachian Trail. When I first heard this statement, I did not understand its meaning. It was not until having hiked about four weeks on the AT that I figured it out. Hopefully, as others hike their hike, they, too, will find their understanding of the statement as well.

> *"It is easier to prepare when you know what to expect."*
>
> **Dr. Fix-it**

Chapter 5
What to Expect on the Trail

What to Expect

When I first started hiking the AT, I was not sure just what to expect. One of the first things I noticed was how everybody was so friendly and helpful. It was a rare instance when I met hikers who wanted to keep solely to themselves. The second thing I noticed was how much stuff some people carried while other people seemed to be getting by with a lot less. In addition to these two items, here are my observations of things I came to expect while on the AT.

- Hiking the AT will be much harder than expected as proven by the low completion rate.

- A rough first week, an easier second week, and by week four, your *hiker legs* will develop and carry you happily along the trail.

- Hiking the AT changes people. I suppose everybody is changed to different degrees, but people change. One of the major differences I learned is just how little or how few things one needs to live. I could now be a minimalist and be very happy provided I had WIFI.

- The AT will be well marked with 2" by 6" white blazes. Having the GPS App *Guthook* on your cell phone along with one of the trail guides will take away the need for maps. You will want to carry an extra battery for your cell phone in case it runs down before you can recharge it.

- Rain. And more rain. It is east to get discouraged; the sun will come out. Suddenly, things will not seem so bad.

- Everybody has opinions about gear and methods. Sort through it all and decide for yourself.

- Expect to have foot and knee problems, both during and after a long-distance hike. Some problems can take months to heal, even after you are through with your hike.

- Some hikers will make their hike an opportunity to party and party hard. Do not expect to see these hikers at the end of the trail.

- Some people care less about personal hygiene than others.

- The more a person cares about personal hygiene, the more people seem to hang around.

- The first week on the trail, the five-second rule applies to food dropped on the ground.

- The second week on the trail, the five-second rule becomes the ten-second rule.

- After a month on the trail, the ten-second rule becomes the "well if you are not going to eat that, . . ." rule.

- Do not expect to shake hands with anyone. Instead, offer to "fist bump" or "elbow bump" instead. When a handshake is proper, extend your fist or elbow, and the other person should respond in kind. This is done to help prevent the spread of Norovirus, a flu-like sickness that can be spread by handshakes.

Expected Trail Etiquette

- The first item of trail etiquette one should remember to avoid leaving any trace of having been there. "Take only pictures, leave only footprints."

- Always stay on the trail and do not bushwhack.

- Camp in designated campsites. If spending the night along the trail, commonly called stealth camping, select a site at least 200 feet off the trail and away from water sources. When leaving in the morning, "fluff up" any vegetation that was damaged. The AT goes across lands managed by different organizations or agencies, each of which can have different regulations regarding camping. What is acceptable in one place is not allowed in another. Keep your eyes open for postings along the trail.

- Build fires only in designated and pre-established fire rings.

- Using privies when possible for bowel movements. Otherwise, dig a cathole 200 feet (70 steps) off the trail and away from water sources. A cathole needs to be 6 to 8 inches deep to bury feces. Toilet paper is supposed to be carried out and disposed of in a trash receptacle. Peeing in the woods is preferred over using privies as urine kills the bacteria that break down the solid waste. Pee at least 20 feet from the trail and 200 feet away from water sources.

Expected Hiking Etiquette:

- When hiking, the person going uphill has the right of way. However, I always try to step off the side even if going uphill just to be courteous. Give the right of way to groups so several people do not have to stop and get off the trail just so one person can pass.

- Occasionally along the trail, people will leave coolers of cold drinks and sacks of snacks for hikers. Sometimes there will be folks who set out a food spread, cook burgers and hot dogs specifically for people hiking the trail. These experiences are called *Trail Magic*. It is OK to take as much as you are offered if you are told to do so. However, when there are limited trail magic items, take one item and leave the rest for others.

- Always speak to others you meet on the trail, even if it is just a quick greeting.

Expected Shelter Etiquette:

- Room in shelters is to be available on a first come, first served basis. Do not save space for hikers that have not arrived. Hikers are to take only enough space for their sleeping pad and sleeping bag. Packs are hung on nails or pegs if provided. Otherwise, they can be stored at a hiker's feet. NOTE: In severe weather, try to accommodate as many hikers as possible.

- When staying at shelters, either in the shelter or a tent site close by, respect others by observing "Hiker Midnight." Hiker Midnight means when the sun goes down, it is time to be quiet and even go to bed. Thru-hikers will be tired and will want to sleep.

- Using the red (or green) light on headlamps will make others happy vs. using white light.

- When listening to music, use earphones.

- When arriving at a shelter after dark or when leaving before dawn, try to keep as quiet as possible.

- If hiking with a dog, use a tent or hammock.

Expected Town Etiquette:

In recent history, some hikers have behaved in such a way that people who used to support hikers have decided to stop. Just a few can ruin things for the many.

Town etiquette simply calls for hikers to be respectful and courteous. If a store has a sign that says, "Please no backpacks inside," then either leave your backpack outside or do not go in the store. If a restaurant says, "Hikers welcome in the back," then go around to the back or move on. When leaving a town, try to be a hiker that the local people either do not remember or if they do, be known as "that hiker that was nice to have around."

Expected Trail Name Etiquette:

Many people, affiliated with or who hike the AT, end up using a trail name. The use of trail names started back in the 1970's when CB radios were popular, and people chose to use a *handle* instead of their name. Handles allowed people to remain anonymous for several reasons, one of which was the fear the Federal Communication Commission would discover someone violating one of the many regulations governing the use of CB radios. By staying anonymous, this fear was diminished.

Trail names on the AT keep with the desire to remain anonymous, but many hikers end up sharing their real names and contact information with other hikers they get to know on the trail. Many stay in contact through social media, both while on the trail as well as after hiking the AT.

There are no *official* rules for trail names. However, there are three generally accepted guidelines:

- Many people do not want to pick their trail name but wait for someone or a group of hikers to give them one. When offered a trail name, hikers can reject it by simply not using it.

- Trail names should have some meaning, a reason for the name, and a story behind the name. A story behind a name gives hikers an opportunity to share about themselves when asked how they got their trail name. Having a story behind a trail name is the reason one should avoid doing anything stupid on the trail before being given a trail name.

- Trail names can be changed by other hikers or by the hiker him/herself.

My original trail name was given to me the first night I was on the trail. I fixed a cooking stove for one hiker, a trekking pole for another, and a tent zipper for a third. They all asked where I learned to do these things, and I simply said I had two degrees in industrial technology as well as always wanting to learn how mechanical things worked. They gave me the name Fix-it Man because they said most thru-hikers had broken gear and when hearing my name, they might ask what I fixed, and could I help them.

Later, I met AT hiker Ohio Grass Man who needed a pot stand and windscreen. All we had to work with was a Monster drink can. When I got it completed, I had made a combination pot stand and windscreen that was awesome. Worked like a champion! Ohio Grass Man said, "You are more than a Mister.

You are a Doctor. I'm changing your name to Dr. Fix-it!" And so, I am now Dr. Fix-it.

So, what all has Dr. Fix-it repaired on the trail? Everything from trail gear to real estate contracts to relationships. I also started "fixing it" when people do not have a trail name. When I discover someone does not have a trail name, I ask if they want one. If they do, I gather any other hikers around, and we listen as the person tells us about themselves, what has happened to them on the trail, and so on. I try to make sure they have several names from which to pick, so they can choose one they like. We keep going until the hiker is satisfied. Here are some of the ones I can remember I have given:

- C Sharp: Musician, played guitar on the trail. I gave him the choice of that or D Flat.
- Ironman: A tall, well built, retired state highway trooper. He shuttles people and close to where he lives is a metal "Ironman" statue. He and his wife run the Rock 'n Sole Hostel.
- Look Out: Hiking with his mother, Tumble Foot, and was always looking out for her.
- On Hold: Put his life on hold to hike the AT. Married to Time Out.
- Tent Stake: Forgot to bring any silverware so for the first thirty miles of the trail, had to eat his food with a tent stake.
- Time Out: Took time out her life to hike the AT. Married to On Hold.
- Tumble Foot: Kept stumbling on the trail. Mother of Look Out.

> *"If you want advice, it has often best to ask people who have been there, done that, and have the T-shirt."*
>
> **Dr. Fix-it**

Chapter 6
Advice from the Trail

During my AT hikes, I took the time to interview over 125 people who self-identified as seniors. While there was not much scientific about these interviews, it was interesting to see how the responses were similar.

When I stopped to visit with a hiker that seemed around my age, I told them about my research and book. I asked them if they would like to help me with my research. Every person I asked to help, agreed.

The first thing I told them that to take part in the survey, they had to self-identify as being a senior. I told them for my study, a senior was one who has had enough life experiences to know what they wanted out of life, and two, were old enough not really to care what other people thought. So, with that as criteria to take part, I asked them this question, "Please give me three bits of advice for people wanting to enjoy the AT." Below are the top ten responses in the order most mentioned.

1. Slow down

This answer overwhelmed all the other answers to my survey. It was as if it would be impossible to enjoy the AT unless one took the time to enjoy it. To thru-hike the AT, the window of opportunity to complete the hike with somewhat decent weather limits the amount of time available to complete the hike. It is reasonable to assume this is a major reason so many also picked "Section hiking is better than thru-hiking."

I started my hiking career when I retired. As I mentioned in the introduction, the first hike I did was a rim-to-rim across the Grand Canyon. I entered the campground lottery and won six nights of camping below the canyon. The only reason I did not spend any more time in the canyon than six days is that is as long as the National Park Service will allow someone to spend below the canyon at one time. I figured if I was going to spend all that time and money just to get to and from the canyon, I needed to spend as much time as possible below the rim. When I reached the top of the south rim, I was somewhat sad that my adventure had come to an end.

During the first morning of my canyon hike, a young man ran around me on the trail. I yelled, "Where is the fire?" He responded, "I'm doing a rim-to-rim today!" To this, I yelled back, "Too bad you won't get to see the canyon!"

In looking back at this experience, I suppose the young man did the right thing if he wanted to say he had run across the Grand Canyon in one day. I hope he does not believe he has seen the Grand Canyon. As I hiked the northern section of the AT, just south of the Mount Katahdin, I met several hikers finishing their thru-hike. For the most part, they all seemed to be glad it was about over. They were doing nothing but hiking north with their heads down, barely wanting to talk to anybody. All business, nothing else. Personally, when I finish something, I want to have enjoyed it enough that I am sad for it to come to an end. I enjoy section hiking because I am sad when my hike comes to an end. If I did a true thru-hike of the AT, I too, would probably be happy when it was over.

2. Section hiking is better than thru-hiking

When I started what I had planned to be a thru-hike, I had every intention of hiking the entire AT in six to seven months. It was just a few days into the hike that I realized I felt like I was an employee of the trail. It was like the boss would be there at the end of the day to see how many miles I had gone. I saw quarterly reviews coming up when I had to be at a certain place on the trail by a certain date if I was to complete this project by the drop-dead date dictated by the onslaught of wintry weather. This feeling was not fun!

GAIL HINSHAW

I went home after 500 plus miles to let my feet and hands heal up. Ten weeks later, I was able to return to the trail, but by then I had lost the window of opportunity to complete a thru-hike that year. I decided to hike until I was ready to come home. This time I realized I was the boss! I could hike as far as I wanted to and then stop. I could take a day off if I wanted. I could spend time visiting with people; I could linger at a shelter. It felt wonderful. The burden of time and miles were gone. I was in charge of my hike, my life. I was the boss!

Because this item was the second most often mentioned piece of advice given by seniors, it obviously should carry much weight in planning an AT adventure. In fact, one senior said during our discussion if a person is planning to hike the AT, then consider a thru-hike. But if a person plans to enjoy the AT, consider section hiking.

3. There is more to hiking the trail than hiking the trail

The AT is not just about hiking, it is about adventure, exuberance, forgiving, healing, accomplishments, history, relationships, nature, spiritual growth, experiencing life to its fullest! It's about being in the moment, living life on the edge, the anticipation of what is around the next bend or atop the next mountain. Regardless of the specifics, all these bits of advice boil down to one thing: There is more to hiking the trail than hiking the trail.

4. The less you carry, the happier you will be

One of the lessons I learned from hiking the AT is good, lightweight equipment will not get you to Katahdin. However, poor, heavy equipment can keep you from Katahdin. When I started my original hike in the middle of the AT at Harpers Ferry, my base weight was around 16 pounds. By the time I added food, water, and stove fuel, I was somewhere from 25 to 30 pounds, which I thought would be fine. Five hundred and fifty miles later, the bottoms of my feet were numb, the area where my toes attached to my foot was so sore, I could not let my toes touch the ground without hurting. Also, my fingers and hands had started to get numb as well. It was time to head home to heal.

When I returned to the trail ten weeks later, my pack was lighter, and my shoes were designed for people with foot problems. In the words of Dana Kee, 2017 thru-hiker, "The less I carry, the happier I am."

5. Hike your own hike and be flexible

The phrase, "Hike Your Own Hike" (HYOH) is often used to encourage people to hike the trail in the way which best suits them, their abilities, and their goals without regard for how others might suggest the task be accomplished. It means for people to hike their speed, to stop when and where they want. In other words, to simply do their own thing. If people follow the expected general guidelines (such as leave no trace), follow standard trail etiquette, and remain situationally aware, all should be fine when you HYOH. If there is one overriding theme of this book, it is Hike Your Own Hike.

6. Use trekking poles

The use of trekking poles has gained in popularity over the past few years. Studies have shown trekking poles take a considerable amount of weight and pressure off the legs and knees (particularly going downhill) as well as putting the arms and upper body to use during hiking. Their use does not stop here. By adding two additional contact points to the ground, trekking poles can help reduce the number of slips and falls. They are useful in checking the depth of bogs and streams, mud puddles, and other hazards. Pack weight can be saved when using trekking poles to erect tents. AND, they can be used as a defensive weapon if ever needed.

7. Document your journey by writing a journal and taking pictures of people as well as places

It dawned on me how important this would be as I grew older once several seniors mentioned this suggestion. One senior explained it this way:

> Taking pictures of a mountain that will still be there in a thousand years is okay, but that picture can still be taken in a thousand years. Taking pictures of the people you meet, the people who help you, the people who make you laugh, is a once in a lifetime opportunity. When you grow old, you will look back at your people pictures, and that will bring you joy.

8. Take care of your lower legs and feet

This one is very personal to me. Within the first 1,800 miles of hiking the AT, I had to leave the trail four times because of lower leg problems. First, it was exercised induced peripheral neuropathy, and then tendonitis; I was afraid it was a stress fracture. This was followed by shin splints and finally, plantar fasciitis. Common denominators in these medical conditions are they all have to do with the feet, and they are the reasons I had to stop my AT hike and go home to heal. Another common denominator is they all seemed to occur after I had hiked 400 to 550 miles. Later, after hiking 1,800 miles, did I learn if I had changed out my shoes every 400 to 500 miles, I probably would have had a good chance in doing a thru-hike. Better late than never, I have been told.

Did I have any other foot problems? Not really, unless three small blisters and a minor sprained foot are what you want to call problems. The blisters received treatment the day I got them. The minor foot sprain received a few strips of tape for a couple of days.

Knees are another potential problem area for hikers. Today, close to five million Americans are living with total knee replacements. The number of knee replacements says that knees are subject to serious problems if not babied to some extent. Hikers who want to take care of their knees will do well to carry as light a pack as possible, start their hike with short hikes, and increase their weekly mileage no more than 10% a week, use trekking poles, and use some knee support brace as appropriate.

No matter how you hike the AT, the experience will not be enjoyable if your feet or knees hurt. Therefore, plan from the start to take care of them.

9. Listen to your body

The number one response to *Slow Down* partly drives this point of advice. However, simply slowing down will not solve this problem by itself. In fact, hikers often told me that by the time they listened to their body, it was too late. For example, an older hiker told me about one of his daughters who years before thru-hiked the AT and put in big miles. It was not until after her hike was complete that she started experiencing knee problems, problems she was still fighting five years later.

Hike today in a way you can enjoy hiking tomorrow.

One hiker told me people should "Hike today in a way you can enjoy hiking tomorrow." Many examples could be tied back to this statement. I once stopped at a shelter before noon because of heavy rain. Another hiker stopped by but then took out in the rain as he felt he needed to keep hiking to get his miles in that day. The next day I passed this same hiker who was taking the day off to dry out his equipment that had gotten wet.

I saw people who would hike for an extremely long day but then take the following day off because they were simply too tired to continue.

Listen to your body also relates to energy levels. One day I would realize I was struggling with not having any energy. Another day I felt like I could conquer the world. Finally, I realized that after I ate lunch, I seemed to have more energy. I decided the problem must be what and how much I was eating. I started to track my food and beverage consumptions. I started researching trail nutrition and soon realized the fuel I put in my tank was driving my energy level. From that point on, I listened to my body about energy levels and adjusted my eating and fluid intake accordingly. This topic is so important, I have included an entire chapter on "Trail Nutrition."

10. Watch the weather

The weather forecasting in existence today is fairly accurate. Weather radar can even give almost minute by minute weather information. The only problem is how to get the weather information while hiking the trail. If cell service is available, this problem becomes nonexistent with the use of today's smartphones. Because there are parts of the trail where cell service is lacking, it is always best to check the weather several days in advance whenever cell service is available. AT weather and weather radar apps are available for download to smartphones. Check the list of resources in the Appendix for these apps as well as other important resources for the AT hiker.

Please note there are parts of the AT that the weather can be extremely dangerous as it can change quickly. Generally, these areas are at the higher elevations of the trail, primarily in the Smoky Mountains, the White Mountains, and on into Maine. Naturally, Mount Katahdin is included in the areas to be especially cautious of the weather.

> **"If you don't know where you are going, any direction or strategy will work"**
>
> Adapted from the Cheshire Cat, *Alice's Adventures in Wonderland*

Chapter 7

Hiking Strategies for the Appalachian Trail

There are several different strategies to hiking the AT. Many things will influence the hiking strategy chosen, including weather, the physical condition of the hiker, time available to hike, finances, and yearning to hike with others or to seek solitude. The north end of the AT is at the top of Mount Katahdin in Baxter State Park, Maine. October 15 is generally when the mountain will close because of severe weather. Some years the weather may force an earlier closure. Hikers wanting to summit Mount Katahdin at the end of their hike should plan on October 1 as a deadline. Those hikers wishing to begin at the north end of the AT should plan to begin no earlier than the first of June to allow the snow to melt on Mount Katahdin. Most hikers will start at the southern end of the AT sometime between mid-February to April 1. This will allow enough time to arrive at Mount Katahdin by October 1. Because of this weather-driven window, a bubble of northbound hikers to develop. This bubble may be fun for those wanting to socialize, party, and be surrounded by people. It also means shelter space, camping spots, shuttles, motels, restaurants, and other services hikers need will be stretched thin. People and businesses may simply be too busy to properly handle the entire hiker bubble. However, for many hikers, this may not be their desired hiking environment, and they should choose a hiking strategy that avoids this herd of hikers.

Conventional Hiking Strategies

There are four conventional ways of hiking the AT, three of which are considered thru-hiking or hiking the entire trail within one year.

Northbound or NoBo Thru-Hike

The most common way to thru-hike the AT is called Northbound or NoBo which is to hike from the south end at Springer Mountain, Georgia and finish at Mount Katahdin in Maine.

Southbound or SoBo Thru-Hike

The least popular method to hike the AT in one year is called Southbound or Sobo which is to hike from the north end at Mount Katahdin and end at Springer Mountain. The reason this direction is not as popular is that you must hike the hardest part of the trail first and will need to start later in the year because of lingering snow in the northern mountains.

Flip-Flop, Both-Bound or BoBo Thru-Hike

An increasingly popular method to thru-hike the AT is called a Flip-Flop or BoBo (Both Bound) and consists of hiking the trail in a non-continuous method. Some Flip-Floppers start from the south end but realize they won't reach Katahdin before it closes due to weather so will jump north, re-start at Katahdin and head back south to the point they left to jump north. Others will simply start somewhere in the middle, head north and after summiting Katahdin, return to their starting point and head south to Springer Mountain. Harpers Ferry, West Virginia and Pawling, New York, are common starting points for Flip-Floppers because public transportation is readily available at these locations. In 2017, Roanoke, Virginia became a train stop for Amtrak. This stop will also become a common starting point for Flip-Floppers. However, the availability of shuttle services allows for many options along the trail that would make flip-flopping starting points.

Section Hiking or multi-day hiking (not a thru-hike)

The fourth strategy of hiking the entire AT is to hike the trail in sections and is not considered Thru-Hiking if it takes more than a year from start to finish. People who are unable to take five to seven months out of their lives at one time or within a twelve-month stretch but want to hike the entire trail may choose this method. This group must be admired if they complete their hike, even when it takes several years to do so. I was privileged to meet one section hiker completing his AT hike after hiking one week a year for 25 years!

Strategy Selection

The strategy selected will have a significant impact on the chance of completing a thru-hike. History tells us that only one in five hikers that start at the south end and head north will complete their hike. About one in three hikers that start at the north end and head south will complete their hike. While this may seem contradictory to this hiking direction being so hard, many believe it is because once these southbound hikers get the hardest part of the trail completed, they know the trail will be much easier for the rest of their hike. However, more than one in two hikers that do a flip-flop thru-hike will be successful.

There are several reasons for the significantly higher success rate of flip-floppers. First, these hikers start in the middle where the hiking is easiest, and therefore, their bodies get in shape before the going gets very strenuous. Second, by the time the hiking does get strenuous, they have figured out what gear they need and have given up carrying unnecessary gear, so their packs are lighter when the hiking gets tougher. They get to hike in better weather. They can avoid the bug season in the north, the mud season in Vermont, and the hot weather in the south and mid-section. They can start later in the spring and then hike later into the fall. They get to hike north with the spring and south with the fall, especially if they head north from the middle around Harpers Ferry, West Virginia, then return to their starting point after completing the northern half and head south to complete their thru-hike.

There is one other enormous difference in a northern direction Flip-Flop hike started in the middle of the trail — these hikers avoid being in the hiker bubble.

Unconventional Hiking Strategy

Thru-hikers try to backpack the entire trail in a year. They carry their camping gear and several days of food every day. Naturally, the further a person hikes, the more likely they are to try to eliminate as much weight from their pack as possible. One way to drop the most weight is not to backpack at all but to do a series of day hikes, often called slackpacking or as I prefer to call it, day hiking.

What makes this a practical option to hike the AT is, as I have stated before, a road crosses the AT an average of every four miles. Except for the 70 miles through The Smoky Mountains National, one can day hike the entire AT. This encompasses only one-third of one percent (.33%) of the entire trail. There are a few places, especially in the White Mountains, a day hike may be longer than one would want to do, but other than these few places, slackpacking or day hiking is possible. It is even possible to day hike the 100-mile wilderness in Maine.

With the advent of more and more hostels along the trail, competition is becoming stiff between the different hostels. As a result, to get hikers to spend more than one night at their hostel, hostel owners have started to offer day hiking options. They shuttle hikers to the trail close to their hostel. Hikers only carry a daypack to a predetermined pickup point at which time they are picked up and returned to the hostel for another night. As the number of hostels along the AT increases, more of the trail can be day hiked using these shuttle services. Day hiking allows for enjoyment without all the pain. Almost all thru-hikers employ day hiking at some time during their hike.

People who call themselves purists or traditionalists believe one must carry all their gear the entire way. However, these same people use modern equipment made from today's modern materials and embrace digital technology on their thru-hikes. I propose day hiking is simply an enhanced method of hiking just as modern materials are an enhancement of equipment. All that said, I have come to believe purists are simply people who think everybody needs to hike the way they hike.

Around 95% of the AT is close to civilization, and with the eastern portion of the United States heavily populated, the AT is constantly crossing roads and highways. The frequent road crossings, many with associated trailhead parking lots, allow for hikers to schedule day hikes from trailhead to trailhead carrying only the equipment dictated by the trail and weather. A simple daypack containing a smartphone with applications including GPS and trail map, compass, weather radar, camera, clock, PDF files of trail guidebooks, and a flashlight is sufficient for communications and trail navigation. Also, a headlamp, lunch, and snacks should be included in the daypack along with water, a method of purifying water, toilet paper, rain jacket, small first aid kit, signal whistle, a backup battery for the cell phone, and any added clothing needed due to potential bad weather. By grabbing this daypack and a set of trekking poles while wearing appropriate clothing, all a hiker now needs to do is to arrange how to start and end the day's hike.

The general problem with day hiking is the need for transportation to and from the trail. The names of hostels and hotels that provide this service along with shuttle companies and individuals can be found in the various hiking guides and websites listed in the Appendix under resources.

Another problem with day hiking is the cost to hire a shuttle driver twice a day, pay for a place to sleep at night and then eat at restaurants twice a day. Some people have spent $20,000 hiking the AT in this way. Two books telling about day hiking are *The Slack Packers Guide to Hiking the Appalachian Trail* by Lelia Vann and Greg Reck and

46 | P a g e

The Don's Brother Method by Mike Stephens. While both books are good reads about how these folks' day hiked the AT, reading these books shows just how logistic intensive as well as expensive it is to try to day hike the AT. However, there is an easier way to day hike the AT as explained in the section entitled Dr. Fix-it's Revolutionary Self Double-Shuttle that is in the next chapter. This method uses only one vehicle and simply needs from two to four people working together as they all hike in the same direction, car camping at night, buying food in bulk to save money, and having extra clothes and gear available as the weather changes. Hiking does not get any sweeter than this!

> *"Every major problem I've had on the AT was caused by not having a vehicle."*
>
> **Two Step, 2017 AT Thru-Hiker**

Chapter 8

Using Shuttle or Trail Vehicles

Conventional Use of Trail Vehicles

One of the easiest methods of day hiking is to use your own vehicle(s) to drive to and from the trail. By having your own vehicle, you have a moving storage shed to keep a variety of items readily obtainable. You can have access to excess food, equipment, supplies, tools and anything else that you chose to have available. The ideal vehicle can also serve as a sleeping shelter. The sleeping shelter vehicle can be as elaborate as a recreational vehicle or as simple as a mini-van. If you do not want to sleep in the vehicle, then a car or pickup would suffice.

The vehicle is positioned at a trailhead, and then you either hike away from the vehicle and arrange for transportation back to your car or park your car vehicle down the trail, arrange for transportation back to the trail and hike towards your vehicle. NOTE: Hiking towards a vehicle is always better than trying to arrange a time to meet a shuttle driver. You can arrive anytime, day or night, and your parked vehicle will be there.

Two people, one vehicle with a Key Swap

If hiking with a partner, a twist on using a vehicle without the use of outside transportation is called a key swap. One person starts hiking down the trail while the other person drives ahead, parks the vehicle at a trailhead and heads back towards the first person. This location can just be one day's hike away which would allow for day hiking or several days away which would require carrying a conventional backpack load. The two hikers then meet in the middle, and the key is exchanged or swapped. In reality, each hiker should carry a key. This way if the hikers should miss each other, no actual harm occurs if the hiker headed toward the vehicle knows where to find it and has a key or knows where the key is hidden on the outside of the vehicle.

Two people, two vehicles

If two people want to hike together and do not want to mess with shuttle services, then two vehicles can be utilized, leaving one vehicle to hike towards and the other vehicle is driven and left at the start of the hike. Once again, these two vehicles could be as close as one day's hike or a hike lasting several days.

One person, one vehicle and scooter/motorcycle/bicycle

If only one person is hiking and wants to avoid using shuttle services, two options are available. The first involves using a vehicle with a scooter or motorcycle, and scooter or motorcycle carrier mounted on the back. The vehicle gets positioned up the trail, and the scooter is used to go back to the starting point for that day's hike. When arriving at the vehicle, the hiker drives back and picks up the scooter and then drives ahead and repeats the process.

One person, two vehicles

One final method of one-person hiking and not utilizing shuttle services requires two separate vehicles, each placed at one end of the part of the trail to be hiked. Pay attention as this gets a little more complicated. In this example, the hiker wants to hike in a northern direction but must hike each day going south to make this method of hiking work. Starting at the northern vehicle, the person hikes south to the vehicle parked at the south end of the part of the trail hiked. The hiker then gets to the southern vehicle and drives to the northern end of the next section of trail to be hiked. The hiker then hikes south till they reach the other vehicle and the process of leapfrogging vehicles continues as the hiker moves north on the trail while day hiking south. If one of the vehicles is outfitted for sleeping, then the hiker can sleep in that vehicle each night.

Dr. Fix-It's Revolutionary "Self Double-Shuttle" Day Hiking Technique

This technique virtually eliminates the need for outside shuttle services while utilizing only one vehicle and two to four people working together while all hiking in the same direction!

Over the years, many techniques have been developed to day hike or slackpack the trail. All the methods I could find relied on coordinating with non-hikers or shuttle drivers; requires the use of two shuttle or trail vehicles, or makes people hike in two different directions. Some of these ways can get very expensive as well. None of these appealed to me. I wanted to day hike but wanted to use only one vehicle. I did not want to spend a lot of money or deal with the expense or coordination of outside shuttle services, and I wanted all participants to hike in the same direction. Day hiking in his way, nobody would complain as who gets to hike downhill versus uphill. Because of my desires, I developed a theory about how two or more people could shuttle each other with only one vehicle. Before I said much to other people, however, I wanted to try it out to make sure I was not crazy. Here is a short story about how the technique was perfected and proven a practical method of hiking.

I had parked my trail vehicle at Uncle Johnny's Hostel in Erwin, TN. I was completing a multi-day hike, heading to Uncle Johnny's and my van. About two miles before reaching my destination, a couple caught up with me on the trail. We visited as we hiked, and I realized this couple needed my shuttling method, and I could use their help in proving my hiking method would work. Dana and Jennifer Kee, trail names of Atlas and Matchmaker, now entered my life.

As we hiked toward Uncle Johnny's, they told me they had started from Georgia, but Jennifer was having problems with her knees and was afraid she might not be able to continue hiking. Dana was wanting to fulfill his longtime dream of hiking the AT. I told them if they would join me for dinner, I would make them an offer they could not refuse.

We soon arrived at Uncle Johnny's hostel, and I introduced them to Letty, my trail vehicle. When they discovered I had a vehicle, Dana said, "You have a vehicle, and you are hiking the AT?"

"Looks like it. In fact, let me show you what is inside." With that, I opened the side door, reached in, and pulled out of the ice chest, two ice-cold bottles of Gatorade. "Anybody want a Gatorade," I asked? With eyes as wide as the tail itself, they nodded in amazement.

Matchmaker said, "Your vehicle even has a trail name?"

I then explained that some thru-hikers told me it was bad karma to have a vehicle on the AT without the vehicle having a trail name. These thru-hikers then proceeded to discuss the situation for an hour or so and decided my vehicle should be named Letty. It stood for **Light at the End of The Tunnel**. From then on, it was Letty who was always waiting for me at a trailhead like a *Light at the End of The Tunnel!*

We then went to the store at Uncle Johnny's for them to check in and for me to arrange to get a shower. As we headed back to Letty where we had left our packs, they asked why I did not have to pay for my shower. "Simple," I responded, "I fixed one of their washing machines and several water leaks in their shower building last week when I left Letty. The manager seems to still appreciate Dr. Fix-it." Such is part of the life of a hiker with a trail name like Dr. Fix-it.

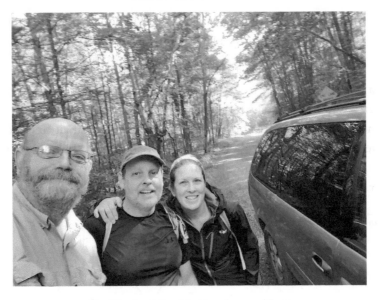

Dr. Fix-it, Atlas, Matchmaker, and Letty

After getting cleaned up, the three of us went to dinner where we got better acquainted. I then explained my idea as a way they could keep hiking and hopefully overcome Jennifer's knee problems. I told Dana and Jennifer they needed to take the next day off and let Jennifer rest knees, put ice on them and take some ibuprofen. I said I was going to give them their key to my van and for them to go to a store to resupply, wash their clothes at a downtown laundry, (washers and dryers at hostels are notoriously busy), and whatever else they wanted to do. All I asked was for them to meet me at 5:00 o'clock tomorrow afternoon at a trailhead called Beauty Spot, about 12 miles up the trail. I was going to leave my pack in the van and day hike to that trailhead. After looking at our GPS software and saw the road that ran to the Beauty Spot trailhead, they agreed it looked like a doable plan.

The next morning, I started my 12-mile day hike to the agreed trailhead. When I arrived at 4:30 that afternoon, Dana and Jennifer were pulling into the parking lot. Dana got out, opened Letty's side door, reached in, and pulled out an ice-cold Yoohoo drink for me, direct from the ice chest they had re-stocked. I think I made the right choice with this couple. We went back to Uncle Johnny's Hostel, got cleaned up and that night we all enjoyed a great Italian dinner.

The next morning, after breakfast at Duncan Donuts, I took Dana and Jennifer back to Uncle Johnny's Hostel. They left their packs in Letty and started day hiking toward Beauty Spot with only their lunches, raincoats, water bottles, water filter, and a small first aid kit. In their pockets were their smartphones, loaded with trail guides, GPS software, and my phone number in case we needed to text or call each other.

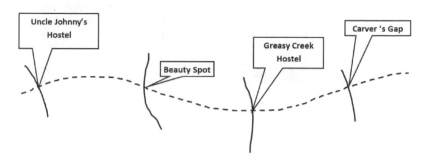

I drove back to the Beauty Spot trailhead and parking lot where I left Letty. I then day hiked on to Greasy Creek Hostel, another 13 miles up the trail. When Dana and Jennifer got to Beauty Spot, they drove to Greasy Creek to meet me. We enjoyed the evening with others at this great hostel.

The next morning, I drove them back to the Beauty Spot trailhead where they got off the trail the prior afternoon, and they started their day hike to Greasy Creek Hostel. I returned to the hostel where I parked Letty. Donning my daypack, I headed up the trail to Carver's Gap trailhead, another 12-mile hike, where I would be picked up once again by Dana and Jennifer and handed another ice-cold Yoohoo.

Two hundred, fifty miles and several cases of ice-cold Yoohoo later, the various nuances of the Self Double-Shuttle were worked out. I had arrived at the place I had left the trail the year before. I had to return home to handle some personal business, so we said our goodbyes and the Kee's returned to normal hiking. The break from carrying a regular pack had allowed Jennifer's knees to heal and the Self Double-Shuttle was now a proven method to hike the AT. Thank you, Atlas and Matchmaker, for your contributions that will help more people enjoy their AT experience and to fulfill their AT hiking dreams.

Atlas and Matchmaker went on to fulfill their AT hiking dream on December 6, 2017, but not until they hooked back up with Dr. Fix-it after I returned to the trail. I was honored to summit Mount Katahdin with my now, life-long friends.

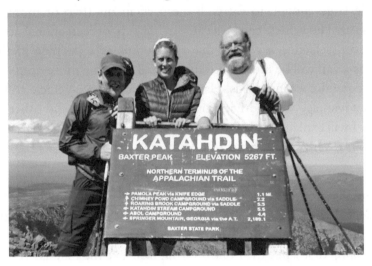

Picture of Atlas, Matchmaker and Dr. Fix-it on Mount Katahdin

I should note that later in their hike, Atlas and Matchmaker decided they would get their own trail vehicle. When they left their Texas home to hike the AT, they were in the process of converting a Mercedes Benz Sprinter van into an RV. This would make an excellent trail vehicle, so they flew home to bring back their own van. Matchmaker decided she would not hike the entire trail but would support Atlas along with others who were thru-hiking the AT. When I joined them to hike Mount Katahdin and head south on the trail, they introduced me to THOR, their trail vehicle. THOR stood for **T**hru-**H**iker **O**mni **R**elief vehicle. They told me it was bad Karma to have a trail vehicle without a trail name. I had heard that somewhere before.

As mentioned earlier, there are at least two published works on day hiking or slackpacking the AT. They provide day by day accounts of how people slackpacked the AT, giving names and locations to various shuttle drivers and trailheads. After reading these accounts, you will realize the logistical nightmare and huge expense it would be to try to day hike the AT, relying on outside shuttle drivers. How much simpler and cheaper it is for two to four hikers to work together to use the Self Double-Shuttle Technique explained in this chapter.

The Self Double-Shuttle day hiking technique only needs one vehicle large enough to carry all the participants (two or more) and their gear. The vehicle can be a car, van, pickup, or recreational vehicle. However, selecting a vehicle that can double as a sleeping platform such as a van will be more enjoyable as well as giving more options for sleeping and cooking meals. Having a high clearance vehicle will also be an advantage when driving on forest service roads and other back roads. I will explain in a later chapter why I chose a 2007 Dodge Grand Caravan for my trail vehicle.

The Self Double-Shuttle starts with dividing the participants into two hiking groups I will call the Lead Group and the Follow Group. Please realize each group only needs one person in the group, but there must be at least one vehicle driver in each group. The Lead Group will start hiking first while the Follow Group will take the first day off from hiking, putting them hiking one day behind the Lead Group. If the two units have different hiking speeds, the faster hiker(s) should be in the Follow Group. This will reduce the time spent by the Lead Group waiting on the Follow Group to pick them up. The Follow Group also requires people with navigation skills needed to find trailheads that are sometimes on back roads and forest service roads.

After forming the two groups, the only decision that needs to be made before the groups split up each morning is the location of the trailhead where the Lead Group will stop hiking and will be picked up by the Follow Group. Trailheads selected must have vehicle parking. Factors to consider when planning the day's hike include how far the groups desire to hike each day as well as the trailheads available.

The basic principle behind the Self Double-Shuttle is the Lead Group hikes the trail one day ahead of the Follow Group. By hiking a day ahead, the Lead Group can drive the Follow Group to their starting point in the morning, then driving the trail vehicle back to the Lead Group's starting point. This is where the Lead Group starts their day's hike up the trail and is the same location where the Follow Group will end their day's hike. The trail vehicle is positioned for the Follow Group to arrive at that evening. The Follow Group can then take the vehicle up the trail to where the Lead Group will be finishing their day hike. This process is repeated each day with the Lead Group taking the Follow Group back to the trailhead where the Follow Group got off the trail the evening before. The Lead Group then drives the trail vehicle back to where they got off the evening before and parks the vehicle so that it will be waiting for the Follow Group that evening. All this allows for both groups to enjoy day hiking without trying to coordinate with outside shuttle services.

To help illustrate the Self Double-Shuttle, let us start by reviewing a normal day of using the Self Double-Shuttle. The diagram below shows four trailheads, each a day's hike apart, labeled A, B, C, and D.

On a normal hiking day, the Lead Group drops off the Follow Group at trailhead A, drives to trailhead B and parks the trail vehicle. The Follow Group hikes towards the vehicle at trailhead B while the Lead Group hikes to trailhead C. At the end of the hiking day, the

Follow Group is at trailhead B with the trail vehicle. They drive to trailhead C and pick up the Lead Group.

The next day, the Lead Group takes the Follow Group back to trailhead B and drives to trailhead C and leaves the vehicle there for the Follow Group. The Lead Group then hikes towards trailhead D to be picked up at the end of the hiking day.

Basically, the Lead Group shuttles the Follow Group in the morning and the Follow Group shuttles the Lead Group in the evening. Evenings and mornings are spent together at anyplace available, be it a hotel, hostel, campground, or even car camping at a trailhead. Naturally, meals can be from restaurants or cooked at a camping site. With the availability of an ice chest, fresh foods are a daily reality, and Dana's ice cold YooHoo's are nothing but unadulterated bliss.

Now that I have explained the basic Self Double-Shuttle technique, I will explain how to start day hiking from Springer Mountain using the technique. The first four trailheads for this example that will be the start-stop points for the hike are shown below on the map. The miles from Springer Mountain are shown in parentheses.

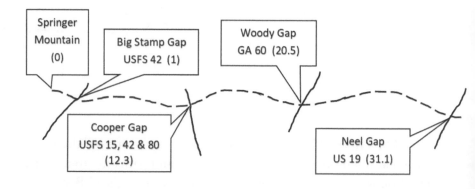

The shuttling process starts with both groups driving to Big Stamp Gap, a mile from the southern terminus of the Appalachian Trail. Everybody hikes the mile to the beginning of the AT, takes pictures, signs the log book, and then all hike back to the trail vehicle. The Lead Group then day hikes to Cooper Gap, Junction USFS 15, 42 and 80, at mile 12.3 on the AT. The Follow Group does not hike anymore this day but drives to Cooper Gap at an agreed upon time later in the day to pick up the Lead Group.

After eating dinner, spending the night somewhere, and finishing off a good breakfast the next morning, the Lead Group drives the Follow Group back to Big Stamp Gap and then drives to Cooper Gap and parks the vehicle. The Lead Group, then day hikes to Woody Gap and the Follow Group, hikes over the same trail that the Lead Group did the day before and arrives at Cooper Gap where the trail vehicle is parked. When the Follow Group reaches Cooper Gap, they drive the vehicle to Woody Gap and pick up the Lead Group.

The next morning, the Lead Group drives the Follow Group back to Cooper Gap then returns to Woody Gap, leaving the vehicle and starts hiking to Neel Gap. At the end of the hiking day, the Follow Group arrives at Woody Gap and takes the vehicle to Neel Gap to pick up the Lead Group. On this third day of hiking, the Lead Group went from Woody Gap, where they left the trail vehicle, to Neel Gap where they are to be picked up by the Follow Group later in the day. When the Follow Group reaches Woody Gap, they drive the vehicle to Neel Gap and pick up the Lead Group.

In summary, every day the Lead Group shuttles the Follow Group to their starting point each morning, and the Follow Group picks up the Lead Group at the end of the day. This process can continue for most of the AT except for the Smoky Mountains National Park and perhaps limited other places that may require a longer day hike than the groups may desire.

Nuances of the Self Double-Shuttle day hiking technique that need an outside shuttle driver.

To help explain the nuances of the Self Double-Shuttle, we will start with the diagram below showing four trailheads, each a day apart, labeled A, B, C, and D.

Use this Self Double-Shuttle technique when there is acceptable road access, but there is no place to park a vehicle close to the trail access. In the illustration above, there is no parking available at B, so a shuttle driver will need to be hired.

The day starts as normal with the Lead Group dropping off the Follow Group at trailhead A, but instead of driving to site B with no parking where they were picked up the evening before, the Lead Group drives the shuttle vehicle to trailhead C. They then call for a shuttle driver to take them back to site B. The Lead Group then hikes to trailhead C and the trail vehicle. The Lead Group then drives back to site B and picks up the Follow Group.

The distance between trailheads will take longer than one day to hike.

This is the situation in the Smoky Mountains National Park. As shown below, the distance from Fontana Dam and Newfound Gap is a three-day hike. The distance from Newfound Gap to Standing Bear Farm is also a three-day hike.

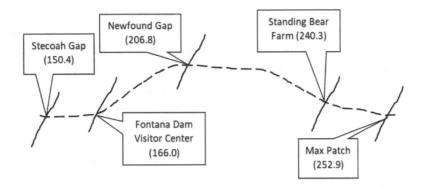

The day starts as normal with the Lead Group dropping off the Follow Group at Stecoah Gap and drives to the Fontana Dam Visitor Center and leaves the vehicle for the Follow Group to arrive there at the end of the hiking day. The Lead Group now starts a three-day hike to Newfound Gap, carrying full packs.

At the end of the hiking day, the Follow Group arrives at the Fontana Dam Visitor Center. The next morning, the Follow Group drives to Newfound Gap and drops off the trail vehicle and hires a shuttle driver to take them back to the Fontana Dam Visitor Center where they start a three-day hike to Newfound Gap, carrying full packs.

After three days of hiking, the Lead Group arrives at Newfound Gap and the trail vehicle. They get cleaned up, resupply, and leave the shuttle vehicle there for the Follow Group. The Lead Group then starts a three-day hike with full packs and heads to Standing Bear Farm.

When the Follow Group arrives at Newfound Gap, they move the vehicle to Standing Bear Farm for the Lead Group to have when they arrive in two days. The Follow Group must now hire a shuttle driver to take them back to Newfound Gap where they start a three-day hike with full packs, headed to Standing Bear Farm.

When the Lead Group arrives at Standing Bear Farms, they resupply but leave the trail vehicle there for the Follow Group. The next morning, the Lead Group day hikes to Max Patch where they will be picked up at the end of the hiking day by the Follow Group who arrived earlier at Standing Bear Farm where the vehicle had been parked.

NOTE: The Lead Group could take a zero day at Standing Bear Farm, waiting for the Follow Group. The Follow Group can then take a zero-day while the Lead Group gets ahead by hiking to Max Patch.

The direction of hiking is to be changed.

There may be a time the groups want to change the direction they are hiking, perhaps in order to hike down a huge mountain instead of hiking up.

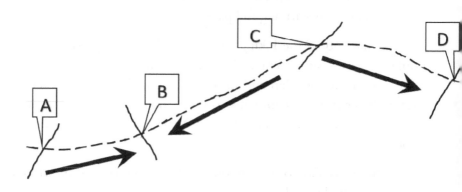

The day starts like normal with the Lead Group dropping off the Follow Group at trailhead A and driving to trailhead B where they leave the vehicle. They then call for a shuttle driver to take them to the top of the mountain at trailhead C, where they hike back down the mountain to trailhead B.

The next morning, the trail vehicle is left at trailhead B, and both groups take a shuttle to trailhead C. The Follow Group day hikes back to the vehicle left at trailhead B. The Lead Group day hikes to trailhead D. At the end of the hiking day, the Follow Group arrives at trailhead

B and the trail vehicle. They then drive to trailhead D and pick up the Lead Group. The following day is a normal Self Double-Shuttle day.

The basic rules of the Self Double-Shuttle include the following:

- Always have one of the groups hiking toward the trail vehicle.

- Always confirm each morning the pickup location for that evening.

- Both groups need cell phones and preferably, satellite communication devices such as the Garman Inreach Satellite Tracker with texting ability.

- If for some reason the Follow Group cannot pick up the Lead Group, they MUST find a shuttle driver to pick up the Lead Group.

- Local people are a great source to verify trailheads and road conditions

Selecting and Outfitting Your Shuttle Vehicle

Are you intrigued by the idea of using a trail vehicle? If so, you need to think about what type of vehicle you need. Just about any vehicle will work provided it will carry all the hikers and their gear. However, some work better than others. When I started working on my method of enjoying the AT, I had limited experience with using a vehicle on the AT. My experience was with Flash 52 who used a Honda Accord. While it worked great as a moving storage shed, where we could store the food and equipment we did not need on the next hike, it did require us to find a place to stay every night. We stayed at hostels, hotels, or car camped.

When I started to look for my trail vehicle, I wanted one that I could sleep in as well as use as a storage shed. It had to be reliable, yet inexpensive. I ended up buying a ten-year-old Dodge Grand Caravan with 125,000 miles. The prior owner had put $3,000 in the front suspension and the engine. I added a new battery, alternator, and new tires. The total bill for this vehicle then came to less than $5,000. Not bad, even though it did have minor body damage, but I figured this just added to the stealth of the vehicle and would make a potential thief think there surely was not much inside to steal. I also thought I would sell the vehicle when I was finished with it and recoup most of my money.

I did black out the back windows with a rubberized, peelable paint available from auto parts retailers that took the already dark windows and made them impossible to see through. I did remove enough of this paint on the two sliding doors that I could see out when driving and allowing people sitting in the back to see out. These openings are covered with clinging, plastic blackout shades when I park. I kept the top of the back window unpainted, so I could see out the top of the back window when driving. I had a large bath towel I hung up behind the front seats when I was camping and when I had to leave Letty parked. I also put a towel over the back window when parking Letty. The towel and the side shades prevented anybody from seeing into the back of the vehicle.

This model had electric sliding doors and Stow and Go seating which allows the seats to be stored below the floor. When the seats are put below the floor, the back is opened up, exposing an area large enough to haul four by eight feet sheets of plywood. I added two plastic chests of drawers I got from Walmart and faced them to the back of the Caravan. I also added a shelf or table that dropped down behind the vehicle and in front of one of the chests of drawers. This allowed me to stand behind the vehicle and in front of the other chest of drawers, all under the back door that when raised up, would protect me from any rain that might be falling. I purchased a folding cot-sized foam mattress for the inside as well as six milk crates for storage that stack up and fit alongside the mattress. The mattress and storage crates all fit between the back of the front seats and the back sides of the plastic chests of drawers. The second row of seats consisted of two bucket seats right behind the front two seats. With these up, I could transport three additional people. When I wanted to sleep in the vehicle, I had to put one of the two back seats down under the floor. I also had room for an ice chest that would keep ice for five days. It was great to come off the trail and enjoy a cold Gatorade as well as give cold drinks to other hikers that were around the vehicle.

This setup allowed me to live up to my trail name of Dr. Fix-it as I carried tools and repair supplies. Over the course of my hike, I was able to help many hikers with repairs, replacement gear and resupply as well as provide shuttle service as appropriate. The one thing I avoided was taking business away from local shuttle drivers who depended upon providing shuttle services for their income.

I later added a new roof-mounted tent for $800. The rooftop tent allowed me to have another person or couple "set up camp" just about any place without looking for an actual campsite. The setup worked especially well at trailheads. I would often go to a hostel, campground, or truck stop and purchase a shower, resupply if needed, purchase dinner and hit the bathroom, then go someplace to set up camp for the night. If the roof tent were needed, I'd go to private or public campgrounds, or stay at a trailhead. If I did not need to use the rooftop tent, I usually slept in a Walmart or hospital parking lot as well as at trailheads.

Having the ice chest allowed me always to have fresh sandwiches and fruit for lunch as well as cold drinks in my water bottles to start my hike each day.

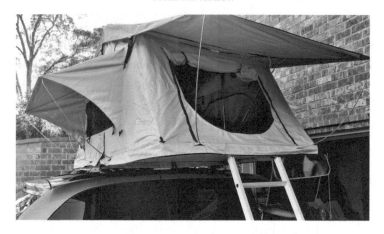

Letty with rooftop tent

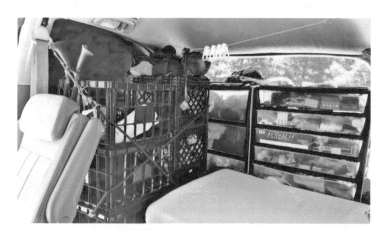

Letty from the inside

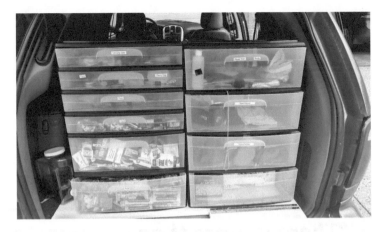

Letty from the back.

> *"There is more than one way to skin a cat."*
>
> **Dads of the world**

Chapter 9

Alternative Ways to Enjoy the Appalachian Trail

There are many ways to enjoy the AT without actually hiking the trail. Some methods involve hiking at least some part of the trail, but other methods allow people to enjoy the AT who cannot hike or even walk. Here are some of the ways some people have enjoyed the AT.

Determine if you are a hiker or camper

Over my years of spending time outdoors, I have come to realize that hikers are different from campers because hiking and camping are two different activities. Backpacking combines the two.

Before you get too far along with planning an AT adventure, it probably would be wise to decide in which category you belong. Doing this early in the planning cycle will help you understand the mental process to use in selecting the strategy about how to best enjoy the AT. I feel that two forces define four distinct categories of people regarding their feeling towards the outdoors. These two forces could be plotted on an X and Y axis graph as shown next.

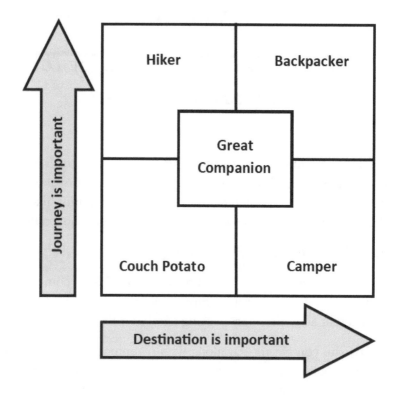

On this graph, the Y-axis represents the strength of the journey is important and the X-axis represents the strength of the destination is important. A person who ranks high on the journey being important but low on the destination being important will fall in the upper left quadrant and labeled a *Hiker.* A person who ranks low on the journey being important but high on the destination as important will be in the lower right quadrant and labeled a *Camper.*

People who rank high on both the journey and the destination is important will be in the upper right quadrant and labeled a *Backpacker.* People who rank low on both the journey and the destination is important will be in the lower left quadrant and labeled a *Couch Potato.* Finally, people who rank around the mid-point of both the journey and destination as being important will be in the middle, able to be happy doing any of the four activities. Therefore, they are *Great Companions.*

Hikers

People who are hikers are those who enjoy the journey. They like seeing new sights, seeing what is around every turn. They are not necessarily into sleeping outdoors but will do it simply to make hiking more doable. Hikers are always looking for ways to reduce what they carry with them when they go hiking. The less they carry, the further they can hike and the more sights they can see. When it is time to stop for the night, they want to set up their tent, eat, and get to bed. People who identify as hikers probably have the best chance to complete an AT thru-hike. They are also the ones most likely to enjoy day-hiking.

Campers

Campers are all about the destination. They are the ones who like to set up camp, start a campfire, put on camp shoes, set out camp stools, and enjoy cooking camp food. They may camp to do other activities such as fishing, hunting, photography, Dutch-oven cooking, or a variety of other outdoor happenings. Campers are always looking for additional camping gadgets to take along on camping trips. If they hike at all, it is simply to get to a campsite. Campers who want to hike the AT will find their packs much larger than the hikers and will probably find that doing a thru-hike of the AT is not going to happen. If they want to hike and camp the entire AT, section hiking may be an option they can enjoy. Or they can day hiking the AT, but with using the Self Double-Shuttle, they get to enjoy car camping in the evenings.

Backpackers

Backpacking combines both hiking and camping. Backpackers carry enough camping equipment to be comfortable but don't overdo it. They will try to lighten their backpacking load but won't sacrifice comfort as they have a certain amount of camper in them. Backpackers' backpacks are larger than Hikers' but smaller than Campers'. If backpackers' bodies hold up and/or they embrace ultra-lightweight backpacking, they have a chance of completing an AT thru-hike. If their bodies don't hold up to conventional backpacking, the Self Double-Shuttle is an attractive alternative as it combines day hiking with evening car camping.

Couch Potatoes

Couch Potatoes are people who find little enjoyment with going someplace, or if they do go, they wish they were not there. Very few Couch Potatoes will probably read this book.

Great Companions!

These people have a balance to their lives. They are not extreme journey people or destination people. However, because they show some interest in both, they can be great companions as they can be happy staying on the couch or traveling someplace. They feel comfortable and enjoy just about any situation; thus, they are Great Companions.

Cherry Pick Hiking

Cherry pick hiking can be hiking the entire trail but different sections of the trail are picked based on the time of the year that is the most enjoyable to hike, or it can simply be hiking only those sections that seem the most desirable to the hiker.

Spot Hiking

Spot hiking is hiking occasional sections of the trail with no intention of ever completing the entire trail. During my time on the trail, I discovered several people and groups that were enjoying the trail in this manner. One senior couple could hike five or six miles at a time. They were simply hiking across one county in Virginia, doing one hike a week. By utilizing two cars, they always had a car at the end of their daily hike. After they completed one county, they then set a goal of hiking across another county. By spot hiking, they never felt overwhelmed.

Another group of senior ladies I met on the trail lived fairly close to the AT. They were section hiking the AT by day hiking and having a driver meet them at the end of the day when they went out to dinner. After dinner, they all went to an inexpensive hotel for the night. They always hiked in the direction that seemed the easiest (generally downhill). After hiking for a few days, they would go home for a week before coming back to hike some more.

One group of ladies I must mention, called themselves "Girls Gone to the Wild." They simply took one day a week and decided where they wanted to hike, drove two vehicles to the trail, and parked at opposite ends of the day's planned hike. Each carload of ladies started hiking toward the other car, met for lunch in the middle, and at the end of the hike, all joined back up for dinner and then drove home.

Experience the AT without hiking the AT

While researching this book, I met an elderly couple hiking the AT in a way many seniors could hike. This couple decided they wanted to experience the AT but being in their eighties, hiking the AT in the traditional sense was not possible for them.

What they did was read several books written by people who had hiked the AT, watched every movie they could find, read up on the history of the AT, followed thru-hikers by reading their blogs, then started out on their own adventure. They started by driving to Georgia and hiking to the top of Springer Mountain from Big Stamp Gap trailhead about a mile from the summit. They then proceeded to drive alongside the AT, stopping at all the places they had read about in the books and seen in the movies. They stopped at restaurants mentioned in the trail guides, talking to and buying meals for thru-hikers. They shuttled hikers back to the trail. They handed out Trail Magic along the trail. They stayed in motels and hostels as they went north, making friends and memories as they went. They even ended up with trail names before they got out of Georgia, but unfortunately, I have forgotten them. They took pictures with hikers and trail angels as well as various business owners, documenting **their** AT Hike. They were making sure to hike a section of the AT in every state, often alongside their new hiking buddies. They planned to continue this until they reached Baxter State Park at the foot of Mount Katahdin where they planned to wait for a group of hiker friends to return from the summit, hopeful of each bringing a small memento rock back to them before taking one last picture as they celebrated their AT Hike.

> *"Anytime a process has an 80% failure rate, the process is wrong."*
>
> **Dr. Fix-it**

Chapter 10

A New Process to Thru-Hike and Enjoy the Appalachian Trail

As I mentioned in the Introduction, in 2017, it is estimated that close to 4,000 people studied, planned, scheduled, and bought equipment to thru-hike the AT. They did all this in the sincere belief they would be successful. Four out of every five of these folks did not complete their thru-hike. Any time a process only has a 20% success rate; the process is wrong. If a failure rate of 80% is unacceptable, then currently the process of how people plan and hike the AT is unacceptable as well. This chapter explains how to change the hiking process to increase the success rate.

Any time a process only has a 20% success rate; the process is wrong.

The current process must be wrong when half of the failed hikers drop out before completing 25% of the trail. What is also interesting to note that according to the Appalachian Trail Conservatory, in recent years, the number of people trying a thru-hike of the AT has been growing while the percentage of people completing their thru-hike is going down. It should also be noted that the people who write books on how to hike the AT are those who are in the small 20% who are successful and because they were successful, believe if others hiked the way they hiked, others would be successful as well. The current failure rate proves this philosophy of hiking is wrong 80% of the time.

The reasons people fail to complete their planned thru-hike are many. While deaths on the AT are extremely rare, injuries are very common and are often the reason given for people dropping off the trail. Even those hikers who are successful, a sizable percentage have lower leg and foot problems for many months following their hike. There is a percentage of hikers who find out that their experience on the AT is not as romantic or as enjoyable as they thought it would be for them. Some hikers get bored. Others simply run out of money or time. Having the wrong clothing and gear can make for an experience that is nothing close to pleasant. For whatever reason people have for failing their quest of thru-hiking the AT, some things can be done to keep people on the trail. This book was written to encourage hikers, and this chapter summarizes what one can do to increase the chance of being in the rare group of hikers who become successful thru-hikers.

Here is a quick summary of the easiest and most pain-free way to thru-hike and enjoy the Appalachian Trail. It is based on the following principles:

- The less weight you carry (within reason), the happier you will be.

- Day hiking is the easiest way to hike and not carry much of weight.

- Utilizing the revolutionary Self Double-Shuttle is logistically the easiest way to day hike and can be the cheapest way to hike the AT.

- Good equipment will not get you to Katahdin, but poor equipment can keep you from it.

- The better the weather, the more enjoyable the hike.

- Avoiding unpleasant situations is a good thing. Unpleasant situations to avoid include the bubble of hikers in the south, the extremely hot weather in the south and mid-Atlantic sections in mid-summer, the mud season in Vermont, and the black fly season in New England.

- The longer the hiking season, the less number of miles must be hiked each day and therefore the less strenuous the hike.

The easiest way to hike the AT is to do mostly day hikes. The easiest and cheapest way to do this is to provide your own shuttle or trail vehicle to get to and from the trail and then use the Self Double-Shuttle. A vehicle you can sleep in is great. Getting a rooftop tent is fantastic if you chose to do the Self Double-Shuttle. Backpacking gear needs to be ultralight weight. Because of using a trail vehicle, gear may be changed out daily when doing the Self Double-Shuttle. Very little gear is needed when day hiking, just watch the weather and adjust gear as needed.

By partnering with one to three other hikers, you will be able to do the Self Double-Shuttle and avoid scheduling shuttle drivers to get you to and from the trail.

Do a Flip-Flop hike, starting at Harpers Ferry and hiking to Katahdin. Then return to Harpers Ferry and hike to Springer. Start around the end of April and attend the Harpers Ferry Flip-Flop Festival kick-off weekend and meet many other hikers doing a Flip-Flop.

An alternative to doing a Flip-Flop from Harpers Ferry is to start at Roanoke, Virginia, approximately 300 miles south of Harpers Ferry on the AT. Because Amtrak started using Roanoke as a stop in 2017, I expect this to become a major starting point for Flip-Flops because being so much farther south than Harpers Ferry. One can start hiking about a month earlier or around the middle of April. This area is past the high elevations of the Smokey Mountains, so winter gear should not be needed. The trail is not too strenuous with only a few high elevation climbs before hitting Shenandoah National Park and easy hiking for a few hundred miles. When one flips back in the fall to go south, there will be 300 miles fewer to hike but by starting earlier, the entire hiking season will be extended by a month. In other words, by starting a flip-flop here, a hiker will have an entire month longer to complete a thru-hike before harsh weather arrives at the southern terminus of the AT.

The advantages of this approach are many, so many in fact that it is estimated that close to three times as many hikers complete their thru-hike as compared to those hikers who start at Springer Mountain. The advantages are as follows:

- The flip-flop method gives the longest hiking season without hiking in too much severe weather. It misses the wintry weather at either end of the trail and the really hot season in the south and up through the mid-Atlantic region. This method avoids the mud season in Vermont, and the Black Fly season in New England. You end up hiking north with the spring and south with the fall.

- Hiking this way starts you hiking in front of the hiker bubble coming from the south and by the time you reach the north end and flip back to the starting point, the northbound bubble has passed altogether.

- The flip-flop method of hiking the AT allows your body to get in shape on the easiest part of the trail, so getting discouraged with a really tough part of the trail will not happen.

- When hitting the toughest part of the trail that is in New Hampshire and Southern Maine, the flip-flopper will be in peak physical shape. Those hikers starting from Springer are often worn down by the time they hit New Hampshire. Those hikers starting at Katahdin must hike the hardest part of the trail before they get in peak shape.

Another way to make hiking the AT more enjoyable is to realize having the correct mental attitude is vital to a successful hike. Having a compelling reason for hiking the AT will help overcome the mental roller coaster ride driven by homesickness, exhaustion, cold, rain, loneliness, illness, rocks, tree roots, steep trails, insects, and an occasional fellow hiker on the trail that is obnoxious. One way to summarize the required mental attitude necessary for a successful thru-hike of the AT is to *Embrace the Suck*. Fortunately, day hiking and the Self Double-Shuttle helps tremendously in this regard by minimizing the suck that needs to be embraced.

One of the major reasons people fail in their thru-hikes is running out of money. If this is a concern for you, consider the fact that the Self Double-Shuttle can be the most inexpensive way to complete an AT thru-hike. This is possible because of the following reasons:

- Up to four people can share the cost of operating the vehicle.

- Backpacking equipment can be cheaper because it will only be used for a few nights and only carried for a few miles.

- Car camping allows for heavy, cheaper, and comfortable camping equipment to be used every night.

- During bad weather, the cost for hostels and hotels can be minimized by car camping in comfort with bigger tents, more comfortable clothing, and other cold weather amenities.

- Food can be purchased in bulk, and the excess stored in the vehicle.

- Meals can be prepared when car camping, so eating out is minimized, and expensive backpacking meals can be avoided.

Use the contents of this book to assist in selecting appropriate gear, food, and clothing to ensure an enjoyable experience on the AT. Study the chapters on the hiking and equipment hacks as well as the chapter on advice from senior hikers. Information in these chapters will allow you to take advantage of what others have learned to make the trail more doable and enjoyable.

Consider a formal training program to prepare for an AT hike. There are several programs designed to help people prepare for an AT hike. However, there is one individual in particular who warrants consideration when it comes to preparing for and hiking the AT. In fact, this person has such a strong record in helping people successfully fulfill their dreams of hiking the AT; he deserves his own chapter in this book. His name is Dr. Warren Doyle, known as the person who has hiked the AT more than any other person by traversing the AT **seventeen** times. His chapter is next.

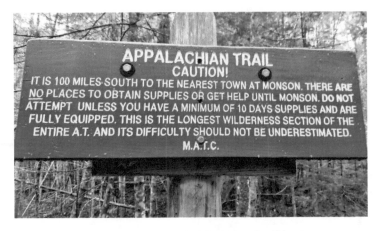

Sign at the northern end of the 100-mile wilderness

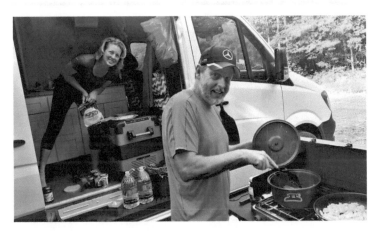

Breakfast in the 100-mile wilderness with THOR vehicle in the background

> *"Better to be a smart hiker than a strong hiker."*
>
> **Dr. Warren Doyle**

Chapter 11

Increasing Your Chance of Success Through Training

The Self Double-Shuttle hiking technique was never intended to be represented as the only way to hike or enjoy the Appalachian Trail. It is, however, intended to be an alternative for those people who enjoy hiking but either do not like camping or carrying the equipment needed to camp in the woods. It is a method that allows hikers who either do not want to or can't carry the equipment necessary to do a conventional AT thru-hike. It can also be used by hikers who need to lighten their pack while they heal from a trail injury. However, there are additional things which increase the chance of having a successful AT experience. And perhaps the best person to know these things is a man recognized as having hiked the AT more times than anyone else, Dr. Warren Doyle.

Dr. Warren Doyle is a retired college professor and has traveled the entire AT a total of seventeen times! He thru-hiked the AT nine times and section hiked it eight times. Based on his vast experience of hiking 36,000 miles on the AT, he has developed several programs to assist people in fulfilling their dreams to enjoy and hike the trail.

Dr. Doyle, being an educator, realizes the importance of training when it comes to being successful. He lives and works 10 miles from the AT, just outside of Damascus, VA. Because of this location, he uses the trail itself as a classroom. He currently offers several programs to budding hikers that are explained on his website, www.warrendoyle.com.

One program is a five-day resident course called The Appalachian Trail Institute (ATI). According to Dr. Doyle's website, www.warrendoyle.com, the program covers "trail history and management, trip logistics, food, equipment, physical conditioning, hiker safety/health; and the most neglected but most important topic of all, the psychological/emotional aspects of long-distance hiking." The website goes on to say ". . . since 1989, several hundred hikers (from thirty-four states and four foreign countries) have attended and enjoyed the ATI."

What I found to be most impressive about the ATI is the 75% successful completion rate for hikers completing the five-day course! Taking this course alone would triple one's chances of success!

Another program offered by Dr. Doyle is his *Smarthike* program which gives trail support for hikers who want to hike the trail during the day but meet up with a support vehicle in the evenings when the hiking group car camps alongside the trail, usually at a trailhead. Smarthike is offered for several sections of the trail.

I would encourage anyone thinking of hiking the AT to at least take the time to research Dr. Doyle's website, www.warrendoyle.com, and determine if one of his programs might be beneficial in either preparing for or actually hiking the Appalachian Trail.

> *"It never bothers me to learn from other people's mistakes."*
>
> **Flash 52, 2015-2016 AT Hiker**

Chapter 12

Hacks to Make Hiking More Enjoyable

This chapter has a variety of hacks and suggestions to make hiking and backpacking more enjoyable. They appear in no particular order.

Hiking uphill help

To make hiking up steep hills easier, shorten your strides by as much as one half. Using shorter strides works like bicyclists shifting to a lower gear to go uphill. Bicyclists keep moving their legs at the same speed, but they simply don't travel as far with each revolution of their legs. When hikers shorten their stride but keep the same speed or rhythm when taking steps, each step does not cover as much horizontal terrain or as much elevation gain as a normal step. Therefore, less energy is required for each step which makes each step easier and more enjoyable.

Determining how far you must hike each day by hiking to *par.*

Par is often defined as a level of reference in value or a level of equality.

To hike to par, you must first determine your *par* miles to hike each day and then keeping track of how many miles are hiked and adjusting the score from par. Hiking to par works if you want to hike the entire AT or simply a section. It lets hikers know how they are doing compared to their plan.

As an example, if a hiker wants to hike the entire AT of 2,190 miles and wants to hike it in 180 days, divide 2190 by 180 to get a par score of 12.17 or rounded to 12 miles a day. If the hiker hikes 10 miles the first day, they are now 2 miles under or below par. On the second day of hiking, if they hike exactly 12 miles, they are still 2 miles under par. If on day three the hiker covers 14 miles, they are now back to par. On day four, if the hiker hikes 15 miles. They are now 3 miles over par. When reaching 12 miles over par, the hiker has earned a day off, called a zero-day, which will put them back to par and right on schedule. By following this simple formula, hikers will always know where they are regarding their schedule. By rounding all mileages to the nearest mile, keeping track of par will be easier, and due to the Law of Offsetting Error, over time your par score will be close.

If a hiker gets ahead of schedule, the extra miles can be set aside to use when the trail gets rough and shorter hikes are required. If for some reason hikers decide to change their completion date, they simply refigure their par for the remaining miles and the remaining days.

Determining if you are on your budget by spending to *par.*

This hack is similar to the one on determining how far a hiker must hike each day and when a zero-day is possible. Determine spending par by dividing the money budget by the number of days expected to complete the hike. The result is the amount of money the hiker has available to spend each day on the trail. On days the hiker stays on the trail, the amount below par grows to allow the hiker to have money to spend when coming to a town. It allows hikers to know if they have *earned* enough money from their budget to stay in a hotel, hostel, upgrade any gear, or must simply resupply food and then hike out of town and camp along the trail.

As an example, if a hiker wants to hike the entire AT on a budget of $4,000 and wants to do it in 180 days, divide $4,000 by 180 to get a daily budget par score of $22.22 or rounded to $22.00 a day. If the hiker hikes for three days without spending any money, they are $66.00 under par (or under budget). If they go to town to resupply, they have this amount of money to spend. Overspending will require them to hit the trail above par by the amount of overspending (or over budget). If they spent less than $66.00, they hit the trail below par by that amount. By following these two simple par formulas, hikers will always know where they are regarding their schedule and their budget.

Hikers can bank money by staying away from towns or stopping only to resupply and perhaps grab a quick shower. This banked money can then be used to enjoy zero days in towns. If for some reason hikers decide to change their completion date, they simply refigure their par for the remaining money and the remaining days.

Cache food and water

Caching food and water might be something to consider when hiking a long distance without being able to resupply. An example might be to cache water on a sweltering day along Little Gap Road at mile 1262.7 in Pennsylvania. This will allow you to have water after climbing up the steep, rocky trail north out of Palmerton, PA. This stretch of the trail goes across an Environmental Protection Agency (EPA) Zinc Pile Superfund Site where the available water is contaminated and should not be used. Caching water can be done simply by stopping where the trail crosses the road and hiding bottled water in the grass along the side of the road. Just don't forget where you hid your cache!

Caching food is a little harder to do. Water in bottles will not be bothered by animals, and the bottles are light so carrying them out is no problem. Food, on the other hand, requires more preparation as well as returning to the cache site to pick up the empty food container. New, unused metal gallon paint cans work well if spray painted on the outside with a camouflage color of some kind. These can easily be hidden off the trail but must either be carried out or picked up later to leave no trash behind. One could also hang a "bear bag" in a tree provided it could be placed out of sight from curious people.

Please note that setting out personal property may be illegal in some places. I never worried about this because I was hiding the property and picking it up later. Besides, I was simply creating my own personal trail magic. However, this did not necessarily make it legal.

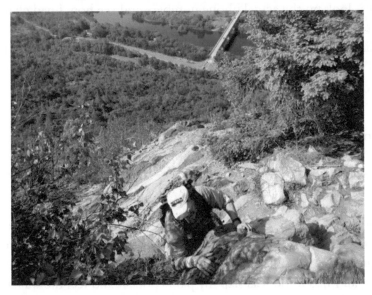

Climbing up trail out of Palmerton, PA. The camera angle makes this photo look pretty crazy. Photograph courtesy of Flash 52

Carrying money and important papers

I am always paranoid when it comes to carrying money and other important papers. To help overcome my paranoia, I first made myself a small wallet from Tyvek material. This wallet was just large enough to carry my driver's license, a debit card, a credit card, a few money bills, a sheet of paper that had a copy of my insurance cards, AARP card, and personal contact information. It also had a door key to my trail vehicle plus a list of all my important numbers, websites, and passwords. The list of important numbers included all bank accounts, credit cards, and hotel and airline mile accounts. I included phone numbers of each to call if I lost a credit card, needed to make a hotel or airplane reservation, or needed help. However, when I created this list, I also created a code that only I knew so if I ever lost this list, no one else would be able to figure out my actual numbers. I applied this code to all the numbers except for the phone numbers. I never changed phone numbers in case someone who was sharp would get my list, look up the actual phone numbers and see how I had changed them and then apply the broken code to the rest of the numbers. Once this list was made, I took a picture of it along with the front and back of all the cards I was carrying, so now I had the information imbedded in my smart cell phone as well.

An example of a possible code would be to take the fourth number in each long number and switching it with the sixth number. This way the number of 123456789 was written on the paper as 123654789.

I also made a small stuff sack out of Dyneema composite fiber material with a drawstring on it. I put my small wallet in the Dyneema stuff sack and attached the drawstring to my pants pocket with a small, locking S-Biner. When I was hiking and started to worry about my wallet, all I had to do was slap my pants pocket and feel the wallet was there and my worries went away. By carrying my wallet on my person, I knew if I lost my pack I would always have my wallet. I also had two, one-hundred-dollar bills hidden inside a re-sealed bandage gauze pad inside my first aid kit just in case I did lose my wallet but still had my pack.

I hid a key on the outside of my trail vehicle, so I could get to it in case I ever lost the key I carried. I also had an extra credit card to another bank, a copy of my important numbers, and a couple hundred dollars hidden away so that if all things failed, I could always buy enough gas to get home.

Keeping your pack weight balanced

While it is important to keep your pack weight as low as possible, it is also helpful to keep the weight balanced as well. A balanced pack allows you to hike standing straight up and not leaning over like hikers with their pack weight only on their backs. A balanced pack is possible by carrying water and other heavy items on a hiker's chest. I carried up to a liter and a half of water on my shoulder straps. This took 3 pounds of weight away from my back and put it on the front. Moving weight from the back to the front causes a shift in the center of gravity of twice the weight shifted. Moving this 3 pounds of water caused a 6-pound shift in the center of gravity which results in walking in a much more normal upright position. See more about carrying water on the chest in the chapter Secrets of Dropping Pack Weight.

Carrying 4 pounds of food on my chest now moved the total weight of the water and food to 7 pounds from my back to my front. This shifted my center of gravity a total of 14 pounds which balanced the weight of my ultralight pack perfectly. See more about how to carry weight on the chest in the next section.

Carry food on the chest

I carried my food on my chest to balance my pack load as well as making snacks readily available throughout the day. I started carrying my food in a DIY pouch that attached to the top of each of my shoulder straps and then attached to the top of my waist belt with two short straps. I had to use these because as I used up the food in my food pouch and drank water from the water bottles hanging on the front of my shoulder straps, my backpack wanted to slip down in the back, and I wanted it to ride up on my shoulders. Attaching the bottom of the DIY pouch to my waist belt solved this problem. The only problem was it was somewhat of a pain to put on my pack and take it off. I later switched to a pack that had a waist belt attached to it, and this is where I then attached the bottom of my food pouch. It was now much easier to handle getting the pack on and off.

After deciding I liked having my pack balanced across my shoulders, I purchased a Z-Packs 4-in-1 Multi-Pack to replace the DIY pouch I had made. It worked like a champ with all the attachment points I needed.

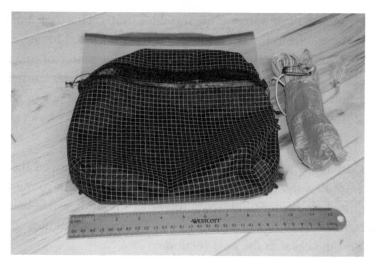

Z-Packs 4-in-1 Multi-Pack

Open all pack pockets when sleeping in a shelter

Shelters are ground zero for problems with mice and rodents. Open all pack pockets so if you have left any food in them, mice will be able to crawl in and eat the food. If food is left behind in a closed pocket, these unwelcome guests will create their own door, and now you will have a hole in your pack.

Use a compactor bag to keep your stuff dry inside your pack AND to blow up your air mattress

A compactor bag works great to line one's backpack to keep things from getting wet from the rain. Also, it can be used as an airbag to inflate an air mattress. I used a NeoAir XLite air mattress. NeoAir sells an AirTap Pump Kit that attaches to a compactor bag to make a pump sack.

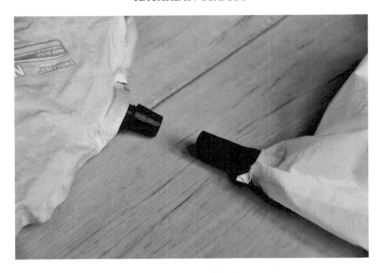

Picture no. 5 of air tap

Throw out your shoes every 500 miles

As hard as it may seem to throw out your hiking shoes that appear perfectly fine, this is what you need to do after hiking approximately 500 miles. The reason for this is twofold. First, your feet and knees must keep working and remain pain-free if you are going to enjoy hiking. Shoes wear out on the inside as well as the outside. When they wear out on the inside, they lose the cushion and support needed to keep feet in a happy state. All three times I had to leave my AT hike because of foot problems was because I did not realize what was happening inside my shoes. They looked good on the outside, but that is not where the cushioning and support originate. Had I changed them out every 400 to 500 miles, I would have had a chance for a thru-hike.

Lace hiking shoes for comfort

Don't assume the normal way to lace shoes is the best way. As I hiked, my feet started to swell, which happens to most hikers. My toes started to get tight in my shoes, and I did nothing to fix the problem.

This pain is what caused me to go home for ten months to heal. Had I known what to do, I could have solved the problem and kept hiking. First, I should have replaced my shoes as they were worn out on the inside, and second, I should have changed how I laced my shoes.

There are several unconventional ways to lace shoes depending upon the problem. In my case where I needed more room for my toes, I later learned to simply remove the laces and re-lace the shoes, starting a couple of holes from the bottom. This reduced my toe pain as my toes were not constricted by the lower part of the shoe. Plus, I still had the shoes tight around my ankle. An internet search will lead you to a dozen diverse ways to lace shoes depending upon a particular foot problem.

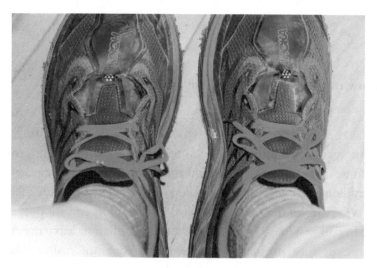

How I laced my shoes to solve my toe pain

Difference between hiking fast vs. far

It has been said if you want to hike fast, hike alone, but if you want to hike far, hike with others. Friendships made on the trail can last a lifetime. Don't lose this opportunity by hiking fast.

Don't carry a trowel to dig cat holes, carry an extra tent stake made from an angle piece of titanium

> ...if you want to hike fast, hike alone, but if you want to hike far, hike with others.

In my effort to minimize my pack weight, I looked for items that could be used for more than one purpose. While I always tried to use a latrine, it was not always possible, and the inevitable poop in the woods was the answer to an immediate need. To properly fulfill this task, a cat hole is dug in the ground about six to eight inches deep and a foot across. Many beginning hikers carry the inexpensive, plastic trowel to complete this task. It does not take long for the trowel to disappear and be replaced with a much more expensive but lighter weight trowel. Instead, I opted to buy a tent stake fabricated from a piece of lightweight titanium angle. This tent stake not only serves as a trowel, but I also had a backup tent stake if I ever needed one.

NOTE: To avoid digging a hole in the dark, while possibly at a time I was in urgent need of one, I would find a spot after I had camp set up and go ahead and dig my cathole. I would often scout a suitable location while looking for a place to hang my food bear bag. By having my cathole pre-dug, it was less of a hassle when the time came to use it.

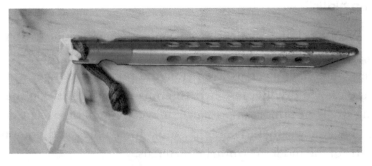

Lightweight titanium tent stake I used in place of carrying a trowel

Attach bright colored surveyor's tape on small, easily lost items

One constant struggle I had when I started backpacking was keeping track of all the various pieces of equipment. One thing I did to help prevent this from occurring was to attach a piece of bright pink surveyor's tape to all my tent stakes, on my knife, and even my car keys. The tape helps me see the items if I drop them or simply lay them down. I never lost a tent stake doing this, but I seldom set up my tent in a campsite that I did not find at least one tent stake someone else had lost.

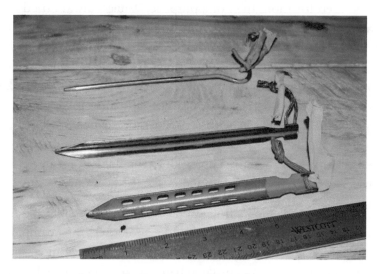

Surveyor's tape on tent stakes

Cotton "kills"

Wearing clothes made from cotton is not a wise thing to do while hiking the AT. Cotton attracts moisture and is very hard to dry. Modern synthetic materials like nylon and polyester can get wet, but they are easy to dry. Because hyperthermia is a real threat on the AT, staying dry is of utmost importance in every condition except during extremely hot weather. Therefore, look for clothes and equipment made from the modern, synthetic materials.

Vitamin "I"

Vitamin I refers to ibuprofen, a common over-the-counter drug used to relieve pain. Because the abuse long-distance hiking does to one's body, aches and pains seem always to haunt hikers. Many hikers use vitamin I on a regular basis. I had an agreement with my wife I would use vitamin I to get over sore muscles, but if I ever got to the point I had to take a painkiller simply to hike, it would be time for me to come home.

"Hire" a Sherpa to carry half your pack weight

I met a beginning, heavy laden hiker that was suffering up Blood Mountain in Georgia towards the beginning of the AT. He was gasping for breath, so I stopped and inquired if he was OK. He just stared back with eyes as wide open as his mouth. His facial expression was one of sheer desperation, so much so he did not verbally respond, obviously not wanting to use the energy required to speak.

I then proceeded to suggest to him if he was planning on thru-hiking the AT, he should hire a Sherpa to carry half his pack weight and that Sherpas were available for only fifty cents a mile. And with that statement, he had caught enough of his breath that we started an interesting discussion.

"You are kidding me," he whispered, trying to save his breath. "Oh, no," I responded. "Only fifty cents a mile to carry half your pack weight. Now the Sherpa wants all his money up front, but you can even put his fee on a credit card if you want. The Sherpa will not only help you the entire length of the AT but will be there for you anytime you go backpacking in the future as well. He will pay all his expenses, so you never have to worry about any additional expense after the initial $1,095 fee."

"You are kidding me," he now exclaimed. "How do I get a Sherpa?"

"It's easier than you can imagine. You simply take $1,095 and replace the gear you are carrying with lighter weight gear plus send home the gear you don't need. You need to learn that you only need about a pound and a half to two pounds of food a day until the next resupply and you need to learn you will only need to carry a liter and a half of water at the most. Once you do these things, it's like having a Sherpa carry half your weight! We are talking a base weight of fewer than ten pounds and a total weight of about twice that at 18 pounds! And after you have hiked a while and have gotten in shape, you can increase your food weight to match your increased hunger."

"I never thought of it like that," he said.

"If you would have lost 15 pounds before you started hiking as I did, then your knees and feet would think as mine think. My legs and feet think I hired a Sherpa to carry all my stuff! And you know what else has happened? My knees and feet now LOVE ME!"

In the Appendix, there is an ultralightweight backpacking gear list that weighs less than ten pounds and costs less than $800. This list is called "Hiring a Sherpa."

The Mental Part of the Trail

Starting an AT thru-hike with a prepared mind can help make a successful experience. Various research studies have shown things a hiker can do to help mentally prepare for a long-distance hike. Some of those things are listed below.

- Don't think of hiking the AT as a 2,200-mile hike.

  If one uses the Self Double-Shuttle, think of the hike as a series of day hikes. If one chooses to backpack the trail, then think of the hike as a series of three to four-day hikes.

- Tell others of your plans to hike the AT.

Potential thru-hikers should tell others of their plan to thru-hike the AT. By doing this, the potential thru-hiker will know that others are cheering them on, so this will mentally help them get through a discouraging time. There will be a feeling of not wanting to let others down.

- Determine why you want to hike the AT; have a purpose or compelling reason.

Knowing why you is hiking the AT will create thoughts that can help you persevere through the tough parts of your hike. Make a list of the reasons you want to hike the AT. Keep this list available to review often. Taking a picture of your list and using it as a wallpaper on your phone will keep it handy to review.

- Create a thirty-second speech that explains why you are hiking the AT.

Having this speech as to why you are hiking the trail makes it easy to explain why you are out on the trail. Always listen as you give your speech to help remind yourself as to why you are hiking the AT.

- Mental toughness can hurt your chances of a successful thru-hike.

Research shows that being mentally tough when hiking the AT is not always good. Hikers will get injured and will need to take time off to heal. People with a high level of mental toughness often try to "hike through" the pain which in turn only gets worse, and these hikers end up not being able to complete their hike. Being willing to stop hiking to heal is critical to finishing the trail.

- Associate yourself with the trail to feel a part of the trail community.

The more a person studies the trail, reads books about the trail, buys T-Shirts, bumper stickers, and books regarding the trail, joins various trail groups, Facebook groups, and in other ways associates themselves with the trail, the more likely the person is to complete their hike.

- Never quit on a harsh weather day.

Never quit on a harsh weather day. When the sun comes out, life will be better, and the likelihood of quitting goes down. Instead, go to town, spend a couple of days thinking about why you are hiking the AT in the first place. Visualize the joy you have experienced along the trail and think about getting back into that feeling. Pick a beautiful day and go back on the trail, refreshed, and thankful you are there.

"Hike today in a way you can enjoy hiking tomorrow."

Extend your daily hiking distance slowly

Too many hikers give up their thru-hike by trying to hike too fast, going too far, carrying too much gear, and doing all this too soon. Start your hike with short days from five to ten miles. Slowly increase this daily mileage by no more than 10% from the prior week. This will allow your body to adjust to the stresses and strains. As I mentioned earlier in the book, one senior hiker told me, "Hike today in a way you can enjoy hiking tomorrow."

Utilize services along the trail

There are businesses and people along the trail who make their living supporting hikers. By using these services, you are helping ensure hikers in years to come will have access to these comforts. As the trail becomes more popular, more amenities will become available. Hostels are growing in number and quality. If you decide to do the Self Double-Shuttle, hostels are a major source of support. If you decide to car camp, they give a place to purchase showers as well as a place to car camp. Most were glad to have me pay for a campsite, even though I was staying in my van and parking in their parking lot. This way I got the advantage of all the other amenities the hostel offered hikers but without having to listen to a chorus of snoring. The folks at hostels are knowledgeable about local trailheads, restaurants, etc. The one thing I avoided was shuttling people with my vehicle. I did not want to take business away from someone who was willing to shuttle hikers.

I have included a list of hostels and hotels in the Appendix of this book. I included those where I enjoyed staying as well as those that carry a formidable reputation among fellow hikers.

Get your picture in the Hiker Yearbook

A former AT thru-hiker named Matthew Odie Norman publishes a Hiker Yearbook every year at the end of the hiking season. Odie has a converted school bus he uses to drive along the AT, meeting hikers and taking their pictures. Odie also has a booth set up at Trail Days. He publishes the Yearbook anually, so hikers can stay in touch after completing their hikes. Odie encourages hikers to send him their picture if he does not get to meet them. Odie can be found on Facebook under his name or The Hiker Yearbook. He also has a webpage at www.hikeryearbook.com.

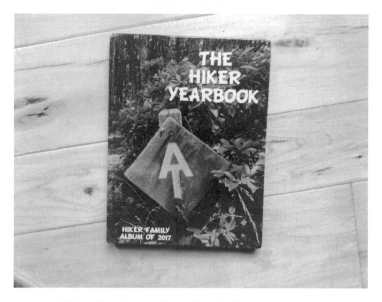

Hiker Yearbook published by Matthew Odie Norman

Things people don't talk about

There are some things people do not talk about regarding hiking the AT. Naturally, religion and politics come to mind. However, here are two additional things that hikers need to know, but few people talk about them.

- Carry a pee bottle or pee bag.

  Pee funnels are available for females to use to make peeing in the woods easier. In the middle of my first night on the trail when nature called, I realized I did not want to get out of bed and go wandering around in the dark, making people think a bear was around. It did not take me long to come up with a solution, thanks to an empty bottle I happened to have with me in the tent. Later, I figured out my great idea was common among thru-hikers.

- Not everybody hangs their food up in a tree.

Lots of hiker's sleep with their food in their tent and seem to get along just fine. If I were going to do this, I would at least put everything that might attract an animal in an odor proof bag. If you are sleeping in a shelter, at least hang your food from one of the "mouse" strings that are in many shelters that keep mice from getting to whatever is hanging from the strings. Otherwise, you can wake up with holes in your pack where a mouse decided to dine on your food.

There are places along the AT where bears are known to cause problems. These areas almost always have bear boxes, bear cables, or bear poles available to properly store anything that might have a smell that would attract wild animals. When any of these items are available, only fools will not avail themselves of their use.

> *"The size of your fears determines the size of your pack. Reduce the size of your fears, and you can reduce the size of your pack."*
>
> **Dr. Fix-it**

Chapter 13
Equipment and Pack Weight

There are lots of books, websites, and YouTube videos about selecting equipment for hiking the Appalachian Trail. I will list some of the better ones in the Appendix under Resources. While this book is about reducing pack weight and day hiking, there will be places on the AT where sleeping out on the trail will be needed. For that reason, I will share a few thoughts about what equipment is needed and how to select that equipment. Please understand, the selection of equipment probably will never stop for me as I continue to enjoy experimenting and playing with backpacking gear.

As a management consultant, I have been asked many times to help people make the right decision about some facet of business. I learned that a person would never know if they made the right decision or not. What they will learn is if they avoided a wrong decision. The same holds true when selecting your equipment. You will never know if you made the right decision, but it will not take long to discover if you made a wrong decision. For this reason, when possible, I always try to buy equipment from sources that will accept returns within a reasonable time.

Because I started my AT hike in the middle of the trail at Harpers Ferry, I did not get to see the circus that happens every spring at Springer Mountain when most hikers start their hike. By the time hikers made it to Harpers Ferry, most had realized that carrying less weight is important to their success in completing their hike. Many of the hikers who drop off the trail before Harpers Ferry never figure this out. The equipment I carried evolved through three basic stages. The first stage was when I started at Harpers Ferry. I felt good that I had my base weight (what my pack weighed, not counting consumables like food, water, fuel, toilet paper, and ibuprofen:) at 16 pounds. I felt I needed to carry about ten pounds of food and a couple of liters of water at about four pounds, so I was carrying a pack that weighed 30 pounds.

...a person's pack is determined by the size of their fears.

As I hiked, I realized I had some items I was not using, so I sent them home. I started carrying food and water based on how far the next town was for food and how far the next water source was down the trail. Even though this approach reduced my pack weight, my body finally broke down at Dalton, Massachusetts after hiking 545 miles. While this weight was considerably less than many hikers I saw the next year when I started to hike at Springer Mountain, it was still too much for me to carry.

My first evaluation of pack weight was when I returned to the trail after a ten-week hiatus to allow my body to heal. It was about this time in my "pack weight dropping evolution" that I realized I started my hike with a pack full of equipment that I felt I needed because of what I was afraid might happen to me on the trail. I began to realize a person's pack size is determined by the size of their fears. I was able to drop pack weight from my original weight by replacing my fears and my pack weight with four things, knowledge, skill, experience, and money.

The first three things, knowledge, skill, and experience were required to calm my fears of what could happen on the AT. The fourth, money, was the simple fact that most lightweight equipment is made from more modern materials which cost more than older materials.

Thru-hikers drop their pack weight as they gain knowledge, skill, and experience on the trail. This is why YouTube videos of gear lists that show what people start with on the trail and what they end up carrying at the end of the trail are so different. I have watched many such videos, and I've never seen a thru-hiker whose pack weighs more at the end of the hike than at the beginning.

When selecting equipment, one can expect to have to make compromises between cost, weight, size, and durability. When selecting backpacking equipment, I have discovered the less something weighs, the more it costs. Buying a heavy tent will cost less than buying a lightweight one of the same size and buying a heavy sleeping bag will cost less than a lightweight sleeping bag that provides the same warmth. Remember, equipment purchases will all be based on compromises. AND, the longer one is going to carry an item, the less cost should play into its selection.

I dropped the weight of my pack itself from 48 ounces to 22 ounces. I also dropped even more items I didn't need; plus, I started to manage my food and water in a much better way. My total pack weight, including consumables, had dropped to around 20 pounds. Plus, I now had a trail vehicle that would make it easier to change out equipment as the need on the trail changed. This made it easier to hike tough stretches of the trail as I would only carry the equipment needed for the next few days until I reached my vehicle.

My second pack weight evolution came when I returned to finish my hike the next year with a base weight of around eight pounds! The pack I carried itself only weighed 7 ounces. I had the same sleeping quilt, but I replaced a bag that covered my air mattress with a custom-made sheet that only fit on the top side at the head end of the air mattress. My shelter weight dropped from 23 ounces to a custom-made shelter of 16.5 ounces. I dropped several ounces of first aid supplies. The next thing I did was work to distribute this weight around my body instead of having it all on my back. I carried 3 pounds with a DIY custom-made hip belt and 5 pounds in my backpack. My food and water were all carried on the front of my pack with the water bottles hanging on my shoulder straps and my food in a chest pack. I never carried over a liter and a half or about 3 pounds of water. My food weighed about 10 ounces a meal. Seven meals would cover me for 3 days of hiking for a weight of 70 ounces, or a little under 4.5

pounds bringing my total carried weight to 15 pounds or about half of what I had started with the year before. It was this gear configuration that had many hikers stopping me and enquiring as to what I was carrying as well as what I was not carrying.

I later changed out my 7-ounce backpack and the DIY hip belt for a Z-Packs Nero pack that weighed the same as these two items but was easier to load in the morning. I did keep the 7-ounce pack for day hiking. The total weight of my day hiking pack with food, water, water filter, backup phone battery, rain equipment, and first aid supplies, was less than 6 pounds.

When I saw the circus at the Springer Mountain with all the beginning hikers, I was the "go to" guy for equipment as well as what to expect on the trail as I had 900 miles of the AT under my belt. I taught people how to use the GPS app on their phone, pitch their tents, hang bear bags, start campfires, operate stoves, and just about any other trail task imaginable. While many were curious about what I had in my pack and many asked me to go through their pack and help them cut some weight (called a shakedown), I soon learned it was a waste of my time. This was because as I have stated earlier, the weight of someone's pack was in direct proportion to the size their fears. Until a person reduced the size of their fears, I could not help them reduce the size of their packs. So instead of giving a person a pack shakedown, we talked about what they feared on the trail. I then tried to share my knowledge as to what was a reasonable fear and what was not.

For example, one hiker had a pack base weight of over 50 pounds. She had three pounds of water filters alone. When I questioned her about this, she was sure she could not hike without them all. She asked me what I had for water filters, and I said I had one that weighed 2.4 ounces. When I showed her my filter, she asked, "Yes, but what are you going to do if you lose it or it breaks?" I said, "Then I would use the water purification pills I carry in my first aid kit." She responded, "But what are you going to do if your filter breaks and you lose your water purification pills?" I responded, "Then I would say, 'Hey, buddy, can I borrow your water filter? Mine broke and I lost my water purification pills.'"

"Ok," she said, "What are you going to do if your water filter breaks, you lose your water purification pills, there is nobody at the creek from whom to borrow a water filter?"

"Well," I said, "if that all would happen, then I would look for a spring that I could get the water right out of the ground and not worry about filtering or treating it."

Then she asked, "What are you going to do if your water filter breaks, you lose your water purification pills, there is nobody at the creek from which to borrow a water filter, AND you cannot find a spring that would be safe?"

"Assuming I don't want to build a fire to boil water, then I would simply hike to the next road crossing and use my cell phone to call for a shuttle driver to take me to town to replace my filter."

"Yes, but what if you did not have cell service on the roadside?" she asked.

My response to this craziness was, "Then I would take out my half an ounce, 20" by 20" piece of Tyvek material I use to put down on wet rocks or logs to protect me when I want to sit down. I use it to protect my knees from mud if needed when getting water from streams; plus, I use it to put at the entrance to my tent to keep mud, rocks, and dirt out. As a last resort, I would take it out of my pocket, unfold it, and hold it up so passing motorists could read my boldly written sign that said, 'Old Hiker Needs Ride.'" This example illustrates how I exchanged knowledge and skill for pack weight.

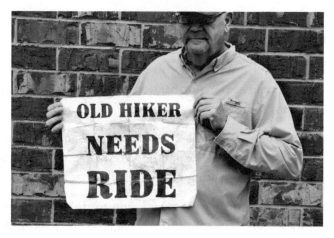

My Tyvek sign I carried for a variety of reasons. It always got a laugh!

Her fears were so big she could not get over carrying a backup filter to her backup filter to her filter. Unable to reduce her pack weight due to her fears, her answer was to go to Walmart and get some pieces of foam to put under her shoulder pads because she hurt so much from the pack straps cutting into her shoulders. I do not think she made it any more than three or four more days on the trail. I also probably do not need to mention there was a hiker who felt the need to carry four knife sharpeners.

I met one young man carrying a sheath knife from his belt that had to be over a foot long and weighing several pounds. When I ask him why he had it, he told me it made him feel safe. My knife is a folding razor blade mounted in a lightweight plastic handle that weighs .3 ounces. This knife works fine, as the only thing I have ever needed a knife for was to open food packages and cut string or cord. Even then, I could always cut cords by holding it on a rock and hitting it with another rock or I could even use my lighter to burn a cord into two pieces. As far as opening food packages, there are probably a dozen ways I could open them when needed. When I wanted a more useful knife, I carried a small Swiss Army knife that still weighed less than one ounce. In addition to a knife blade, it also had a fingernail file, scissors, toothpick, and tweezers.

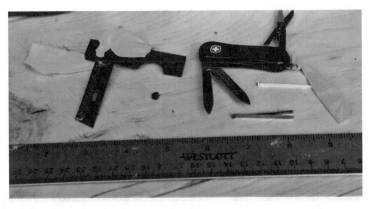

I carried the knife on the left when I day hiked; it weighs .3 ounce. The one on the right weighs 1 ounce, and I carried it backpacking. Both have bight surveyor's tape attached to them so I would not lose them.

> *"The less I carry, the happier I am."*
>
> **Dana Kee, aka Atlas, 2017 Thru-Hiker**

Chapter 14

Secrets of Dropping Pack Weight

There are several secrets to dropping pack weight. Below are some general guidelines when selecting gear. Following the guidelines, is a list of gear broken down into different systems to understand better the equipment needed. General guidelines for selecting equipment are:

- Realize the size of your pack will be in direct proportion to the size of your fears. You must first reduce your fears before you can reduce the size of your pack.

- Reduce your fears with knowledge, skills, and experience.

- The lighter your pack weight, the more enjoyable it will be to carry.

- The more uses for an item, the better.

- Saving the first few pounds is easy, saving the last few ounces gets hard and expensive.

- Don't carry an item that is not needed. As an example, I saw a hiker carrying a 16-ounce canister of fuel when he was going to be out for one night and only cook one dish for dinner. He needed 1 ounce of fuel or less and a much smaller stove as well. If he would eat a cold dinner, the entire cooking setup with stove, fuel, pot, and spoon could be left behind.

- Reading reviews and watching YouTube video reviews will help you decide what equipment will work for you.

- A kitchen-type scale is great to help in selecting the equipment to be carried. A serious hiker knows the weight of everything carried, including what they carry on their person.

Start with Reducing Your Fears

Knowledge, skill, and experience are the keys to reducing your fears. I suggest you increase your knowledge by studying the gear lists I have included in the Appendix and see how I slowly went from a typical hiker to an ultra-light hiker. Other good gear lists, in particular, come from unsupported FKT thru-hikers. These are thru-hikers that try to set new "fastest known times thru-hikes" meaning they are trying to be the fastest person to hike a trail without being supported. These folks strive to reduce not just ounces but grams! Their selection of equipment needs to be studied closely.

The book *Ultralight Backpackin' Tips* by Mike Clelland is a major source of information regarding how to lighten your pack. Clelland has some great ideas. I don't necessarily agree with all his suggestions, but I'm sure he won't agree with all of mine either. One thing we can all agree on is the less we carry, the happier we can be.

Three people to follow on YouTube are *Follow Bigfoot*, *Darwin Onthetrail*, and Dixie on her Youtube channel, *Homemade Wanderlust*. They have some great reviews of equipment and are always looking to improve their gear and techniques of hiking.

Another source to help you gain trail knowledge and reduce your fears is to read trail journals from current and previous hikers. www.TrailJournals.com is a wonderful place to find trail journals from people who have hiked the AT in the past or are currently on the trail. Following people through their trail journals is a great way to get a feel for the trail and what you can expect when you hike the AT.

Once a hiking strategy is determined, the selection of equipment should start. These items are the backpack, sleeping system, and shelter or tent. When determining the equipment you want to use, and especially the bigger and more expensive items, be sure to go online and enjoy watching video reviews plus reading reviews of the assorted options for equipment under consideration. While there are many equipment options available and many opinions expressed, these reviews will help you make an informed choice. Just remember the general guidelines given at the start of this chapter. Check out the Resources listed in the Appendix for additional help in selecting equipment. Also, in the Appendix under the topic, *Hire a Sherpa . . .,* I have included a gear list of lightweight equipment for a tight budget. Using inexpensive equipment is especially good advice if you decide to day hike the AT because you will only be carrying the equipment from 70 to 100 miles. The budget ultralightweight gear list provided in the Appendix costs less than 800 dollars and weighs less than 10 pounds.

Beginner backpackers tend to go overboard on food. The prior chapter explains what I did to overcome my fear of not having enough food. By following the food planning method described, you will be able to overcome your "not enough food" fear and in turn, cut your pack weight substantially.

Backpacking/Hiking System

The first item in the backpacking/hiking system is the backpack. It should probably be selected last to keep from buying a pack the wrong size. Carrying a pack larger than needed will cause excess gear and weight to make its way into the pack. Of all the equipment I carried, my pack caused me the most problems in "getting it right." Here is the list of packs in the order I used them. I did keep the 25-liter, 5.85-ounce pack as my day hiking pack but without the hip belt and chest pack.

75-liter, 48-ounce pack

55-liter, 22-ounce pack

25-liter, 5.85-ounce pack, 5.4-ounce DIY padded belt that carried 2.5 pounds of gear on my hips and a 3.5-liter, 3.25-ounce chest pack

38-liter, 12.2-ounce pack with attached 3.5-liter, 3.25-ounce chest pack

If I had to start over in pack selection, I would start with looking at 40-liter packs that weigh less than 20 ounces.

Sleep System

The sleep system refers to both a sleeping bag or sleeping quilt plus a mattress or pad. Sleeping bags have traditionally been what people used but sleeping quilts are lighter and when paired with an insulated mattress or pad, are just as warm. The mattress or pad needs to be both comfortable and lightweight. When paired with a quilt during cold weather, they must also provide some insulation. Many younger hikers opt for lightweight foam pads, but I carry more weight to have a bigger and more insulated pad because I figure if I am sending from eight to twelve hours on it a day, I want it to be fantastic. I also attach a sheet to the top of the pad since I like to sleep without a t-shirt and I do not like the feel of the air mattress next to my skin. Also, this sheet has strips of Velcro down each side that line up with Velcro on the sides of my sleeping quilt that attaches the quilt to the sheet, eliminating chilly air coming in the sides of my quilt as I sleep. Attaching the down quilt has given me at least 5 to 8 degrees of warmth. I currently use the extra-large size Therm-a-Rest Neo-air air mattress and a Go-Lite 30 degree down quilt.

Go-Lite is out of business, but if I had to replace it, I would look at a quilt from Enlightened Equipment or one from Z-Packs. The air mattress with the sheet weighs 19.75 ounces, and the quilt weighs 21 ounces.

Like I said before when I'm backpacking, I believe the extra comfort I find with this air mattress and sheet is worth the extra weight.

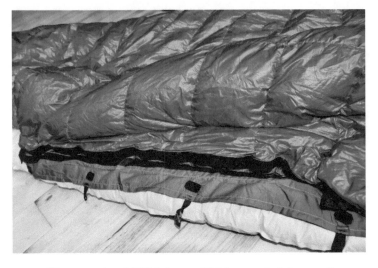

Sleeping pad with DIY sheet and Velcro attached down quilt

Shelter System

A shelter system includes a tent or tarp, tent stakes, poles, and ground cloth. My favorite shelter is a Z-Packs Duplex if I know there are going to be bugs or mabe a lot of rain. My tent with stakes weighs 26.5 ounces. If I know there are no bugs out; I will take my DIY tarp shelter with a raised edge floor (called a bathtub floor) and with stakes, weighs in at 16.5 ounces. Both shelters use my two trekking poles for support.

If looking for a shelter, consider one from Z-Packs if you want the lightest yet roomy tent. If you are trying to save some money, then a shelter from TarpTents or Six Moon Designs would be a great place to start looking.

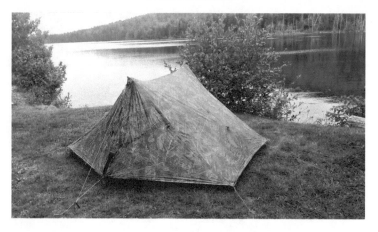

Z-packs duplex tent – 26.5 ounces

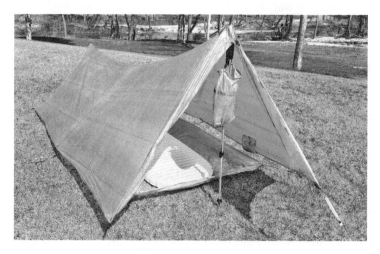

DIY tent – 16.5 ounces

Water/Hydration system

Water is abundant on the AT. For this reason, not as much water needs to be carried as you might expect, except during dry seasons. Water reports are easy to get by asking any hiker coming from the other direction. Be ready to report back on water from the trail behind.

Some people think it is safe to drink directly from the streams and springs along the AT. I never would take that chance as I don't enjoy being sick, and as easy as it is to treat water, it just seems to be the thing to do.

Treating water can be done by filtering, chemically, or boiling. Boiling takes too long and uses too much fuel. That leaves filtering and chemically treating the water. Chemical treatment is the lightest weight, using either a two-part liquid system such as Aquamira Water Treatment Drops that uses chlorine dioxide to kill bacteria and viruses or one of several different water purification tablets. Some hikers use drops of simple chlorine bleach. The tablets are the easiest to use, simply drop a tablet in a water container and then wait appropriately thirty minutes or however long the instructions say. The problem with this system is the required wait time. I like to use a filter system, so I can drink water at once at the water source and then move on. This way, by drinking quite a bit of water at a water source, called *cameling up*, I can carry less water in my water bottles. I always had the chemical tablets with me as a backup water treatment option if my filter failed. I use both methods if the water comes from a pond or a stream that ran through a farm field or pasture. When I used both, I would filter first then treat the water with chemicals.

Filters will eliminate bacteria but not viruses. Viruses are generally not a problem along the AT, so the filters work fine by themselves.

Sawyer brand filters are the most prevalent on the AT. They make two filters, the mini, and the regular squeeze filter. Most minis are soon left behind as they are slow and too hard to use and get replaced with their big brother, the regular Sawyer Squeeze. Both filters utilize either a water bag or a water bottle. Smart Water brand water bottles fit on the Sawyer filters and work well.

Katadyn BeFree Collapsible Water Filters use the same technology as the Sawyer filters but come with an easy to use collapsible water bag. These filters have not been on the market as long as the Sawyer brand, but they seem to be growing in popularity as they are easier to use than the Sawyer filters because of the faster flow rate.

I also like the BeFree because of being able to pack a soft, collapsible bag.

Water is carried in either a water bladder or in water bottles. A heavy-duty water bladder is carried in the backpack with a drinking tube attached that runs up to the face and contains a bite valve on the end from which to drink. This bite valve allows the hiker to have a drink of water at any time without stopping. This feature is very handy, but the drawbacks of the water bladder are many.

The disadvantages of using a water bladder are as follows:

- The heavy weight of water is on the back of the hiker, causing the hiker to bend forward to maintain the center of gravity

- Inability to ascertain water levels

- Not knowing how much water is still available

- Can leak in the pack and get a lot of items wet

- Hard to keep clean

- Hard to get into and out of backpacks

The advantages of using a water bladder are as follows:

- Always having water available to drink, even while hiking

- Can carry a lot of water

Carrying water in lightweight water bottles saves weight, and instead of cleaning the bottles, they simply are replaced. These water bottles are mostly carried on the outside of packs and may require either a buddy's help or the removal of the pack to access the bottles.

By placing water bottles on the shoulder straps with one containing a drinking tube with the bite valve, the ability to always have water available while hiking is exactly like using a water bladder. PLUS, not only can the hiker monitor his/her water intake and remaining water available, others can see this as well. By exposing the water bottles, hikers can monitor the water intake of each other to help prevent dehydration. Because water bottles are readily available on the AT, keeping the bottles clean becomes a non-issue as replacing dirty bottles with clean ones can be done at anyplace water is sold. The tube with bite valve can be cleaned periodically to keep the entire drinking system sanitary and fresh. With the water bottles on the outside of the pack, naturally if one would break, nothing inside the pack can get wet like it can with a water bladder breaking.

Water bottles can be attached directly to the shoulder straps with small carabiners tied to the bottles and then clipped into split rings attached to the shoulder straps, or they may be placed in pockets attached to the shoulder straps. Bottles attached with the carabiners will need to have the bottom secured to the pack straps with small diameter elastic cord to hold the bottles in place. These bottles can either be removed, and the hiker can then drink from them; a drinking tube can be placed in the top of one with a bite valve on the end, so water is available without missing a beat.

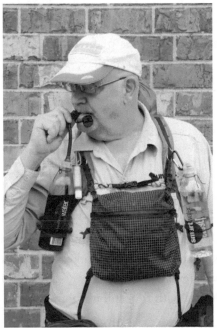

Water bottles and food pack balanced my pack

Cooking System

Most AT thru-hikers only use a cooking system to heat water for their food and to create hot drinks. Hot water is added to dehydrated food and allowed to set for a few minutes. The food can be kept in the plastic bag used to carry it, and hot water is simply added to the bag. The food is then allowed to sit a few minutes to complete the cooking process. Cleanup is simply to put the dirty bag in your trash bag. Another way to cook food is to add the food to the hot water in the metal cup used to heat the water.

A cooking system consists of a stove to heat water, fuel to use with the stove, and a metal container of some kind. Also included in the system is a method of lighting the stove, a windscreen, and an eating utensil of some kind such as a spoon, fork, or a combination spoon and fork called a spork. Some hikers also carry a cozy, or an insulated covering, to put around the plastic bag with the food. This helps retain heat and speeds up the cooking process.

When selecting a cooking system, the first choice to be made is which fuel to use. The five types of fuel normally used are white gas, compressed gas, alcohol, solid tablets, commonly known as Esbit tablets, and finally, wood. These fuels each have their advantages and disadvantages.

White gas stoves and fuel containers are the heaviest type of cooking system and are most often used when a group is cooking together. Therefore, they seldom are used on the AT.

Canisters of compressed gas are next in the weight category but are also the easiest to use and heat water the fastest. It's fairly easy to find this fuel along the trail, but the problem is many hikers don't want to carry two canisters of gas, so most hikers discard the canisters they had been using whenever they buy a new canister. This means many canisters are discarded with fuel still in them.

Alcohol is used by many hikers because it is lightweight and easy to find along the trail. The downside of alcohol is it's a liquid and can spill. Plus, if it spills on something flammable, it can burn! Picnic tables have been destroyed because of burning alcohol being spilled on them.

Esbit Tablets are the lightest weight but the hardest to find along the trail. They are also hard to light, so some hikers carry a small plastic bottle with an ounce or less of alcohol to put a couple of drops on the Esbit Tablet to make it easier to light.

Wood is used one of two ways. Most all camping sites and shelters have a pre-established fire pit or ring. Only a few hikers will build a campfire and use it to cook meals. Most all campfires are built by section hikers as thru-hikers are too tired to worry about a campfire. The second method of using wood to cook is to use a small, lightweight wood burning stove. While a few hikers use these methods to cook, the problem with wood is hikers are tired when coming into camp, and the desire to eat as efficiently as possible removes wood as a fuel source to cook.

There are two alternatives to cooking food. The first is simply a plastic jar with a watertight lid that is used by hikers to put the food in to be rehydrated and eaten. The appropriate amount of water is added to the dehydrated food, and the lid is used to seal the jar. The food is then eaten cold after the food has had time to rehydrate.

Another option is not to carry a cooking system at all but to carry food that requires no cooking. Not cooking makes the evening meal look much like a cold lunch normally eaten on the trail.

The first picture below shows three different types of stoves and their fuel. They include a compressed gas stove, a DIY alcohol stove, and an Esbit tablet stove. The second picture shows a complete cooking system, including a 750 ml pot set on top of an Esbit stove, surrounded by a windscreen. Also, in the picture is a Bic mini lighter, a small bottle of alcohol to put a few drops on the Esbit tablet to make it easier to light, a package of soap leaves, a folding knife, a compressed towel, a spork, and a cozy. The weight of this cooking system is 7 ounces.

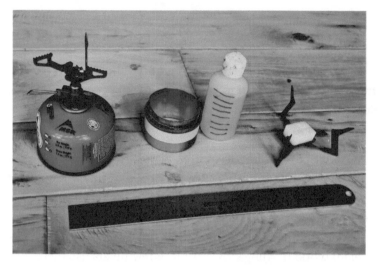

Canister stove, alcohol stove and an Esbit stove

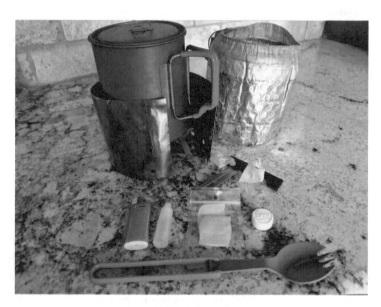

Cooking system that weighs 7 ounces

Food Storage System

The Food System consists of the equipment to carry and store food while hiking/backpacking. Most backpackers use a dedicated food stuff sack often referred to as a "bear bag" which is hung in a tree at night to keep animals from pilfering the food. Most backpackers use a bag from 8 to 15 liters in capacity. Also included in the food system is usually 40 to 50 feet of "bear bag" rope, a small carabiner, and a small bag called a "rock sack." Some systems also include a "smell resistant" plastic bag manufactured by OPSAK that is to keep animals from even knowing the food is around. There is also a company called Ursack that makes storage bags that are marketed as bear proof and other bags that are rodent proof. One final possible part of a food system could be a bear canister that is a heavy-duty plastic container that bears cannot break. Bear canisters are not needed on the AT but are mandatory on some trail in the western part of our country.

What is needed on the AT? Most hikers carry a waterproof food bag and 40 to 50 feet of rope. Few will add the small carabiner to hang their bear bag using what is called the *PCT Bear Bag Hang.* Many hikers simply tie a rock to the end of the rope and use that to launch the rope over a tree limb to raise the food bag. I like to carry a small stuff sack that holds the rope when not in use and then use it to place rocks in instead of trying to tie a rock to the end of the rope. When rocks were not available, I packed dirt in the small bag. Once, I avoided using dirt by simply placing two Snickers Bars in the small bag and used their weight to get the rope over a tree limb.

While I started with a 15-liter bear bag hanging kit from Mountain Laurel Designs, I switched to a chest mounted pack of 3.5 liters. The food for the first day out does not need to fit in the food bag as it is eaten before time to hang the bear bag. When I was going to hike for more than three days, I simply used an additional stuff sack to hold the overflow.

The lightest weight food bag I saw on the AT was one hiker who used the plastic bags that he got to carry his food from the grocery store.

During my time on the AT, I saw about every possible method of storing food at night. The best way to store food was to use the heavy metal Bear Boxes provided at some shelters and campgrounds. These were usually only available in areas where bears have been problematic.

Some backpackers hang their food in a tree while others hang it in the shelter from a rope run through a small can to make it *mouse proof*. Some backpackers simply kept their food with them in their tents. I even saw one hiker put his food up on the roof of the shelter to keep it from bears.

All these methods seem to work fine as far as I could tell. I also hiked 1800 miles on the AT without even seeing a bear. But for me, I used the bear boxes or hung up my food along with anything else that had a smell such as toothpaste, insect repellent, and water bottles that had been used for flavored drinks.

Clothes System

My clothes system consisted of two main parts: the clothes I hiked in and the clothes I carried. I also considered my rain gear to be part of my clothes system as I wore the rain jacket when I was cold even if it was not raining. Between the clothes I wore and carried, I had the following:

Long sleeve shirt with sleeves that could be buttoned up at the elbow

Lightweight T-shirt

Pair of convertible pants with zip off legs (Zipped off legs were carried as weather dictated)

Pair of lightweight running shorts with pockets by Nike

Pair of extremely comfortable underwear

Two pairs of socks, either Darn Tough or Injinji Toe Socks
Ball cap modified to attach a cooling towel around the sides and
    in the back
Neck Buff
Down hood (as weather dictated)
Rain Jacket
Rain Skirt or Kilt

I never had to carry a puffy jacket or sweatshirt. On cold mornings, I put on my T-Shirt, long sleeve shirt, and rain jacket along with underwear, the convertible pants, sometimes with the legs attached but, most times I never bothered with the zip on legs. And of course, socks and shoes completed my attire. I would pack-up as quickly as possible and start hiking without eating breakfast. Within a half mile, I was warm enough to start removing clothes. On cold evenings, I either started putting the layers back on or simply went to bed. I was able to avoid carrying any additional clothing by doing a Flip-Flop hike that kept me out of the really cold weather.

First Aid System

My first aid system included many of the items I started with, but I simply reduced the amount of each item I carried when I finally realized I only needed enough supplies to get me to the next town.

I started my planning for my AT hikes with a visit with my doctor. He had taken the time to study the AT and had a good idea of the medicines I might need on the trail. He phoned the prescriptions to a Walmart Pharmacy, so I could refill any of them I might need while on the trail. Here are the items in my first aid kit after I had hiked 900 miles. They were all carried in a plastic bag. The pills were in a very small, plastic container. The creams were repackaged in small plastic bags.

Prescriptions:

Sleeping Pills for when I simply could not sleep

Medicine for Tendonitis (Added after I got tendonitis)
Antibiotic for Lyme Disease
Liquid Steroid for Poison Ivy

Over the counter medications:
Pepto Bismol pills for stomach problems
Imodium AD for diarrhea
Benadryl pills for allergic reactions and itching
Benadryl cream for itching
Ibuprofen for muscle pain
Deet insecticide
Triple Antibiotic for cuts and sores
Bee Sting Wipes

Blister prevention/repair:
KT Tape
Leukotape Sports Tape
Band-Aids
Second Skin
Duct Tape

General first aid items:
Antiseptic Wipes
One use Super Glue
Mini compressed hand towel
Tweezers
Needle with Dental Floss for Sewing Repairs
Safety pins
Tick Removal Key

Repair/Safety System:
The Repair System items were carried in a watertight plastic bag that also included the first aid kit.
Dyneema Fiber Repair Tape
Duct Tape

Clear Repair Tape for Air Mattress Repair
Rip Stop Repair Tape
Safety Pins
Zip Tie

Misc. Repair/Safety Items:

Repair and safety items were carried with the first aid items.
Mini Compass
Paper Book Matches
Derma-Safe Folding Utility Razor Knife
Waterproof Writing Paper
Ballpoint Pen Refill
10 feet of 1/16" cord
Katadyn Purification Tablets to Backup Water Filter
Black Diamond Ion Headlamp
Thumbnail Size Flashlight
Backup Batteries for Thumb-Sized Flashlight
A piece of Esbit Heat Tab for fire starter

Personal Hygiene System:

The toilet paper was carried in a plastic bag along with the Hand
Soap Leaves. Lip Balm was carried in a pants pocket, and the
toothbrush and toothpaste were carried in the cook kit.
Toothbrush and Toothpaste
Hand Soap Leaves
Toilet Paper

Electronics:

Everything but the inReach Explorer Sattelite Communicator was
carried in a plastic bag, and the InReach was attached to the outside
of my pack.
Recharge Battery for Cell Phone with charging cable
Garmin inReach Explorer Satellite Tracker
Earphones

Rain Protection:

My rain protection system is included in the Clothes System as they were a part of my way of keeping and warm.

> ### *"If you do not need it, why carry it?"*
>
> **Dr. Fix-it**

Chapter 15

Controlling the Weight of Food and Drinks

As I have said earlier in this book, food and water are two things that hikers seem to over pack. Knowing how much water to carry and drink, what food to eat, when to eat, and how much to eat is all part science and part personal preference. Let us start with water.

How much water to drink

Most people never think about how much water they drink. People get thirsty; they get something to drink. Life goes on. However, when doing a heavy exercise like hiking long distances, water becomes of extreme importance. People can go a few weeks without food and survive but can only go just a few days without water. The body is dependent upon water for several things including controlling body temperature, flushing the body of waste products, preventing constipation, and helping perform all major body functions. Most hikers, especially during hot weather, get concerned about not drinking enough water. Many old timers say the easiest way to know if people are drinking enough water is to make sure their urine is clear and not getting dark. Dark urine is supposed to be a sign of not getting enough water.

Drinking too much water, however, can also be dangerous and is called overhydration which can lead to water intoxication. Water intoxication occurs when the amount of salt and other electrolytes become too diluted in the body. The major concern of overhydration is a condition called Hyponatremia— when the salt or sodium levels become out of balance with the water within a body. Death by overhydration is highly unusual, but it can happen.

I found the easiest way to avoid overhydration is always to drink water having electrolytes or consume sports drinks such as Gatorade. The various flavors available can make consuming electrolytes an enjoyable experience. I try to avoid water flavoring that does not have some electrolytes.

The only time I have seen overhydration on the AT was one 70-degree day. I was following a younger hiker who hiked faster than I did, but I would catch up to him whenever I came to a water source as he would be filtering water to drink. The mountain we were on was leaking water about every mile.

I asked this young man, "what's the deal?" He told me he just could not get enough water and was drinking a couple of liters every mile or so. He also told me he was getting light-headed, was feeling weak, and funny as well.

I enquired if he was taking any electrolytes with his water. He told me he never heard of it. I told him that was probably his problem and gave him some Skratch brand hydration mix to put in his water. He drank some as we sat and visited. Over the next hour, he started to feel much better as he continued to consume water with a strong mix of electrolytes.

I always carry water on my pack shoulder strap with a tube and bite valve. This way I can sip water anytime I want. The temperature and how much I am sweating determines just how much water with electrolytes I drink. The amount of water can vary from a liter to two liters every three to four hours.

How much water to carry

I try to avoid carrying any weight I will not need. The amount of water I carried depended upon the weather, the temperature, and the distance to the next reliable water source. The smartphone app *Guthook*, along with the trail guides, show how far the next water source should be. However, as I have said before, I would always verify this by asking hikers I met how far was the next water source.

How Much Food to Eat and Carry

I have said the one thing most people carry too much of is food. I had seen people leave town with a week's worth of food when the next resupply town was only two days down the trail. People carrying a gallon of water when water was available every couple of miles or so on the trail was also a common sight. Why do they carry this extra food and water? It reflects the size of their fears. Once I was day hiking and simply forgot to put in my lunch and snacks. Guess what? I hiked that day, and at the end of the day, I WAS STILL ALIVE! Was I happy? Not at myself for being so stupid that I forgot my lunch which included Lobster Mac and Cheese! Did I ever forget my lunch again? No, but if I had, I would still be alive today.

I realized I needed to cut down on how much food I was carrying when I showed up in town with a bag still full of food. I had carried all that remaining food for several days and over numerous mountains for no good reason. I realized this cowboy was not going to make that mistake again and started by figuring out how much food I needed. And so, started my study of nutritional requirements to hike the long distances.

I knew I needed 3,600 calories a day or 1,200 calories per meal on the trail. If I were burning more than this, either I would lose weight, which I needed to do, or I could plan to make up the difference when I hit town, which is what I did. I wanted to hike into the next resupply town with just a candy bar and maybe a tortilla left in my food bag. I already knew that typical trail food has an average of 115 to 120 calories per ounce. Therefore, I would need an average of 10 ounces of trail food for every meal I was going to eat on the trail. When I went into a grocery store to resupply, I would determine how much food I needed to carry. I then would subtract how much food I already had and buy just enough food to match the weight I needed to carry to the next resupply. As I would shop, I would check the net weights of the food I was buying. I took the calculator on my smartphone and simply added the weights up as I went down the aisles. If I ran out of available weight before I had everything I wanted, then I started the negotiations with myself as to what I wanted most.

As my body got into better shape and needed more calories, I slowly increased the weight of the food I carried but never to the point I had much food left over when I walked into town to resupply or when I reached my vehicle.

Considering what I had learned on the trail about the food I needed to carry, I suggest you start your food planning with buying the most valuable tool in reducing pack weight, a simple kitchen scale. These cost around $20.00.

Put together three days of trail food and water. Note the calories of each food item. Also, set out the fuel you think you will need to prepare the meals you plan on cooking. Weigh each item and get a total weight, including food, water, and the required fuel. For the next three days, eat only the food you have set aside, practice preparing the food, noting the weight of the food, the amount of water you use, and the amount of fuel needed. Keep track of everything consumed. Use only the water you have set aside but use it to make the drinks you are planning to have on the trail such as coffee and hot chocolate. Use only this water to rinse out your cooking pot, brush your teeth, and wash your hands.

Hopefully, at the end of this experiment, you will discover what I learned on the trail, and that is one will need from 2,500 to 3,000 calories a day or around 10 ounces of food per meal. A three-day hike should need lunch and dinner on the first day. The second day will require breakfast, lunch, and dinner, and the final day breakfast and lunch or a total of seven meals for a total of 70 ounces of food. Therefore, there is no need to carry more than 70 ounces of food for a three-day hike, as I learned the hard way while on the trail.

The water used in this experiment should help you learn the amount of water needed each day. Because you will most likely camp close to a water source and cross at least one source of water daily, generally, you should only need to carry one-sixth of the total amount used during the three-day experiment. I learned to check my guidebook and cell phone trail app to know when to expect the next water source. As I have said before, I then I would ask hikers I met about the next water source. I would then be prepared to give them a water report for the trail behind me.

The longer a person hikes, the more the body will start wanting more calories. This is called hiker hunger and is what I experienced when I felt the need for more than 3,000 calories a day. Hiker hunger hits hikers within two to four weeks of hiking and will make you require more food, however, by this time, you will be able to better understand the amount and type food to carry, and the extra weight will not be a big concern.

One way to study how much food to carry is to put the food for each day in its own zip-lock plastic bag. This way, you will eat the right amount of food each day and not have to worry about running out before the next resupply. Also, the first bag emptied can be used as a trash bag. Because these bags are reusable, the bag used for trash can be washed out and used again.

I later figured out that some foods gave me more energy than others, so I started to buy the right mix of foods to give me the most energy. Please see the next chapter on *Nutrition and Energy* to help select what foods to eat on the trail as well as what to eat when going into town. Selecting the right quantity and mix of foods will provide you with the energy to enjoy hiking.

> *"An army marches on its stomach."*
>
> **Napoleon Bonaparte**

Chapter 16
Nutrition and Energy

When I first started long distance hiking, I chose food that was easy to carry and that I enjoyed eating. After a couple of weeks, I discovered some days I could burn up the trail with energy. Other days, I struggled the entire morning. However, after lunch, I almost always felt good with my energy level.

It was at this time; I began to realize just how important food must be to my energy level and in turn, to my enjoyment of hiking. By studying nutrition, it dawned on me that Napoleon was right when he said, "An army marches on its stomach!" This chapter is a summary of what I learned through my study and experience.

There are several considerations when deciding the foods for long distance hiking. Hopefully, the following information will aid in the proper choice of foods for hiking.

Easy to carry

Foods that have a lot of calories in each ounce are known as being calorie dense. Dry foods are easier to carry than foods that contain liquids because of the risk of spills. Dry foods can be repackaged into zip-lock plastic bags and into proper portion sizes that match the amount of food desired. Naturally, cardboard boxed food should be reduced in size by repackaging into plastic bags. Using plastic freezer bags for carrying food will allow for cooking in the bag, provided adding hot water is all that is required.

Large bags of crackers, granola, nuts, and candies, can be repackaged into snack sized plastic bags that are easy to pack.

Easy to fix on the trail

The easiest foods to fix on the trail are those that require no preparation other than opening their package. Any bar fits this category along with dry, loose foods like trail mix, nuts, and chips. Cookies and Pop-Tarts also fit this "easy" category. Great dinner meals can be food that simply needs hot water added and allowed to sit for a while. Cleanup is as easy as dropping the dirty plastic bags into your trash bag. You can wipe your eating utensil clean and then when heating water for the next meal, simply put it in the hot water to sanitize.

Won't spoil

With most foods considered trail foods, spoilage is not a problem provided the food is eaten before the expiration date on the package. Hard cheeses are acceptable but should be eaten early in a hike. When day hiking, most any food can be carried by taking proper precautions. As an example, for lunch, I could enjoy Lobster Mac-n-Cheese from the deli counter available at some grocery stores. I would keep the already prepared meal on ice, and when I left for my day hike, I would wrap the meal in my rain jacket to keep the meal cold. At lunchtime, the food would still be cold.

Subway sandwiches are another food many hikers carry out when leaving town. I have seen many pieces of pizza eaten for lunch as hikers would order more than they could eat when in town and then keep the left-over pieces in their hotel/hostel refrigerator overnight.

Calorie Content

Calories are a unit of measure of energy. Without calories, there is no energy. Our bodies use energy to function, even when remaining motionless. Most female adults need at least 1,200 calories a day to avoid weight loss while male adults need at least 1,800 calories of energy a day to avoid weight loss. People gain weight when they consume more calories than they burn and lose weight when they use or burn more calories than they consume. Estimates show a normal long-distance hiker will use from 4,000 to 6,000 calories of energy every day of hiking. Therefore, to keep from losing weight, this range of calories must be eaten for every day of strenuous hiking. If one is day hiking, the consumption of this number of calories is not a problem as only lunches are carried and then only one lunch at a time. The bulk of the required calories can come from town food or at least prepared when car camping. However, if carrying food for an extended period without any outside food source, then calorie content becomes an issue.

However, you cannot only be concerned about calories alone. Calories come from three main sources, fat, carbohydrates, and protein. Because the body responds differently to each of these sources of calories, foods should be selected based on gaining a proper mix of calorie sources. With today's nutrition labeling standards, determining the source of calories from various foods is simply a matter of learning to read the required nutrition label.

Fats as a Calorie Source

The body uses its fat as a kind of battery to store energy. Any excess energy stored as fat is available when more energy is required than the energy available through food. If more energy is needed than is readily available from stored fat, then muscle can be utilized to provide the energy.

Fat contains about twice the calories of an equal weight of carbohydrates or proteins. Therefore, foods high in fat content are very calorie dense. An example is olive oil. It contains 240 calories per ounce. Nut butters are also very calorie dense with cashew butter having 182 calories per ounce and hazelnut butter with 174 per ounce. Peanut butter is also high in calories with 166 per ounce. These numbers compare to an average of around 115 to 120 calories per ounce for typical trail food.

With fats being so calorie dense, many hikers will add them to other food, such as adding olive oil to pasta, potatoes, rice, and just about any meal that is cooked. And of course, the various nut butters are often consumed spread on tortillas, crackers, bagels, and even eaten directly from the containers.

While at rest, our bodies get up to 60% of the energy we need to sustain life from fat. However, when we get active, the body draws on carbohydrates (which includes sugars) for immediate energy but relies on fat to slowly replenish the energy taken from carbohydrates. Because hiking is at a pace that is comfortable for the body, and not like running which needs energy in a big way, fat can also provide some of the energy along with carbohydrates. When the body has used up all the available carbohydrates, and energy from fat cannot keep up, the body does what is often called hitting the wall. This feeling of premature death is because the body is not very good at quickly turning energy loose from its body fat. What is needed is a quick shot of carbohydrates (i.e., sugar) which is available in the form of a candy bar such as Snickers. (Snickers, by the way, is a staple of food on the AT and is often referred to as the "Breakfast of Champions.")

Carbohydrates or Carbs Content

As previously mentioned, carbohydrates or carbs furnish the body with immediate energy. The body quickly breaks down carbs into glucose or sugar that is sent into the bloodstream. It is then stored in the liver and muscles if not immediately needed to energize the body. It is for this reason that before an athletic event, athletes often do what is called carbo-loading to build up glucose stored in the body.

As the body requires energy, it comes first from glucose in the blood, followed by the glucose stored in the liver and muscles. Once this available stored energy is depleted, the body then turns to trying to get energy from fat stores as well as directly from muscles. As stated in the section above regarding fats as a calorie source, fats can also provide some energy directly when the exercise is at a slower rate such as hiking. If sugar is made available, the body does not have to work as hard to get glucose into the blood system as if it had to make glucose from more complex carbohydrates, such as rice, potatoes, or pasta as well as trying to get it from fat. A review of any quick energy supplement will show a very high concentration of carbohydrates and a sizable percentage of the carbohydrates will be sugars.

Protein Content

The body uses protein to build and repair itself. It is the building block of muscles, bones, skin, and blood. It also helps provides some energy but not in any form that is immediately available. Unlike fats and carbohydrates, proteins are not stored for use later. Proteins are either used by the body or turned into glucose or fat for storage.

Because the body uses proteins to repair muscle and other tissues, it is important to include protein in your diet. Generally speaking, protein powders are easier for the body to digest than proteins from food. Also, foods high in protein are usually also high in fat content that is harder to digest. For this reason, bodybuilders and other athletes will consume protein powders as part of their bodybuilding regiment. Hikers are constantly using and damaging their muscle tissues and therefore need protein to assist in the rebuilding of tissues. Carnation Instant Breakfast protein powders are often used by hikers to get protein in a form that is easy for the body to consume.

Vitamins and other Supplements

There is more to nutrition than just calories, carbs, fats, and proteins. While many people feel they get a benefit from adding vitamins and other supplements to their diet, many have a tough time believing there is any benefit because seldom is the benefit felt immediately. Many people believe eating a balanced diet will provide all the vitamins and minerals needed for good health. However, some say that because of the nature of trail food, a diet of trail food is not a balanced diet. Therefore, the following information is provided as a starting point for people to do their studying and to help determine what vitamins and other supplements should be added to their diet.

Supplement	Form(s)	Benefit
Electrolytes	Liquid, Powder	Electrolytes in the world of nutrition refers to minerals dissolved in one's body fluids that help the body fluids function properly by creating electrically charged ions. The more a person sweats, the more electrolytes are needed as a supplement. Generally taken as powder added to a drink or are in drinks referred to as sport drinks.
Glucosamine, Chondroitin, MSM	Pill	These three supplements are often combined into a single pill that is suppose to promote joint movility and flexibility as well as helping to rebuild cartilage. Available from GNC stores under the trade name of TRiFlex™.
Multipurpose Vitamins	Pill	Multipurpose vitamins generally contain a wide variety of vitamins, minerals that can cover the various vitamin and mineral deficiencies in diets that are not properly balanced.
Probiotics	Pill	Probiotics are the opposite of antibiotics as they are considered friendly bacteria to the body. The body needs probiotics to help with digestion of foods as well as helps the body take in nutrients. They also help the body to prevent being taken over by "bad" bacteria. Particularly useful to reestablish friendly bacteria during and after taking antibiotics.
Vitamin C	Pill, Powder	Vitamin C appears to play an important role in the repair of connective tissues which in turn, decreases recovery time between heavy exercising activities. It also seems to play a role in keeping the immune system functioning at an optimal level. Being a strong antioxidant, it can help reverse body damage caused by free radicals which may interfere with normal body cell function.
Vitamin D	Pill, Powder	Vitamin D has shown to have an effect on muscle pain and weakness. It aids in helping with bone desinity and bone repair, especially in older populations. Research has shown it has a positive effect on athletic performance.
Zinc	Pill, Powder	Zinc is an essential mineral required by the body to grow muscles and ward off illnesses. People on a high carb diet but low on fats and proteins are more likely to need added zinc than people on regular diets.

Planning Your Menu

The body needs calories in the form of carbs, fats, and proteins. According to several sources as well as my own experience, a ratio of 3 grams of carbs to 2 grams of fat to 1 gram of protein seems to be a great starting point in planning a menu that will support a healthy body on a long-distance hike. Remembering how to plan a menu becomes as easy as 3-2-1. The only other breakdown is the amount of sugar in the carbs. The faster one needs the energy; the more sugar one needs in the carbs.

There are several nutritional charts in the Appendix which show the calories and their source of carbs, fats, and protein. The charts are based on one ounce of food, so it is easy to compare the different foods. By studying these charts, one can determine which foods are most beneficial while hiking. There are additional nutritional charts for readily available town food as well. As an example, a McDonald's Big Breakfast with pancakes contains 1,350 calories!

When to Eat

Many long-distance hikers find themselves on the trail for about 10 hours a day with the remaining 14 hours spent in camp. During the day the body needs energy to keep moving, but at night it is time for the body to restore and rejuvenate itself. With this as a basis for eating, the nutritional needs of the body start the day before. One needs to allow the body to absorb the daily nutritional needs in the best way possible. The following is a routine I learned and is easy to follow and works quite well to allow this to happen when on a long hike.

About 30 minutes to an hour before stopping for the evening, eat a trail snack such as a bar or trail mix to kick-start your body in its healing/restoring mode. Taking a probiotic pill at this time will allow it time to dissolve and absorb into the digestive system before the evening meal and will permit your body to more easily absorb the nutrients from the evening meal. When getting to your stopping place for the evening, set up camp then prepare the evening meal that is well balanced but has 40 to 45 percent of the daily calorie needs. With my meal, I would finish taking the vitamins and nutritional supplements for the day. Next, hang or store your bear bag and then crawl into bed. This routine allows your body to slowly absorb the nutrients from the meal over the next ten to twelve hours.

Upon waking in the morning, eat a breakfast that contains plenty of carbs (popular choices include oatmeal with raisins and brown sugar, Pop-Tarts, Honey Buns, or Fruit Pies). If there is a need for added protein, consider Carnation Instant Breakfast mixed into oatmeal. Chew a multivitamin and wash it down with a product called Emergen-C® which has lots of electrolytes, vitamin C plus several of the B vitamins. I would also take my morning allotment of nutritional supplements as well.

The body responds best when it is constantly refueling throughout an exercise activity. Therefore, one thing to consider is eating two lunches a day. After hiking for about three hours, stop for the first lunch. Two to three hours later, stop again for second lunch. Keeping the body refueled on a constant basis will allow the body to be able to continue hiking. An alternative to two lunches is to keep moving but eat something every hour which would produce the same effect of constantly refueling the body.

As the final step in a nutritional routine, look for fruit/vegetable smoothies that are sold in the refrigerated section of the store when you go in to resupply. One national brand is called Naked. Get one made from green vegetables and one made from fruit. These smoothies will help the body get the fruit and the green leafy vegetables it needs. Plus, when eating out, always try to get a green salad and a cup of fruit. Doing these things will give you the needed fresh fruits and vegetables that are too heavy to carry on the trail.

One final thought about nutrition. When in town, eat foods with a lot of protein such as hamburgers as well as some carbs in the form of French Fries! And do not forget the importance of Ben and Jerry's Ice-cream in sustaining a long-distance hiker. The good news is there are only 360 calories per serving of Ben and Jerry's Peanut Butter Cup ice-cream. The better news is there are four servings in a pint of ice-cream, provided you are trying to load up on calories. The sad news is after you have completed your thru-hike, Ben and Jerry's Peanut Butter Cup Ice-cream will still contain 360 calories a serving.

> ## *"Be Prepared."*
> **Boy Scout Moto**

Chapter 17
Trail Safety

Crazy things happen along the Appalachian Trail, things that are unexpected. To keep from being "That Hiker," we need to consider a chapter based on the Boy Scout motto, "Be Prepared."

This chapter is not meant to be a primer on trail safety but instead to point out the potential hazards that can occur during long-distance hiking. The following items are presented for your consideration to stay safe on the trail.

The Ten Essentials

Here is a list of ten items that experts consider to be mandatory when hiking in the backcountry:

Navigation items such as a map and compass
Protection from the sun
Extra Clothing
Headlamp or flashlight
First-aid supplies
Fire building equipment
Repair kit/tools
Extra food
Extra water
Emergency shelter such as a lightweight space blanket, tube tent/garbage bag

Because the AT was so heavily traveled as well as being close to civilization, I did not carry all these items all the time.

Animals

The major animals that can cause problems for hikers on the AT are as follows:

Bears

Most AT thru-hikers see about a half dozen bears on their journey. Fortunately, the bears found along the AT are Black Bears. These bears are seldom aggressive to humans provided they are not provoked or threatened. The National Parks System has created a website that explains what to do if seeing a bear. The information from this website is summarized below:

Respect a bear's space by not getting close to them. One must be especially careful if coming upon a mother bear with cub or cubs. A guideline to know if you are a proper distance from any wild animal is to hold your thumb up in the air at arm's length, and if the animal is completely hidden from sight by your upheld thumb, you are probably a safe distance from the animal. Keeping a distance of at least 200 feet is recommended by authorities at Shenandoah National Park.

Don't advance towards a bear but instead remain still, let the bear know you are a human by talking to the bear in a calm voice and slowly wave your arms. Pick up small children immediately. Move slowly away, preferred sideways. DON'T run away as the bear may give chase. If the bear charges, remain in place, keep talking, slowly wave your arms and pray the bear will stop short.

DO NOT drop your pack as it will help protect your back if attacked. Dropping a pack will also teach a bear that food is in hikers' packs, and, therefore, hikers are to be charged.

Most times when a black bear charges, it turns away at the last minute. This charge is called a bluff. If a black bear does attack, fight back, preferably with kicks and blows to the bear's face and muzzle. NOTE: According to the National Park Service, playing dead is the accepted approach if attacked by a grizzly bear but not by the black bears that are found along the AT.

Ways to avoid bears include hiking in groups as this creates noise and a larger human smell. Groups also appear larger to bears and, therefore, should be of greater fear to the bear. Talking or singing while hiking in bear country will, hopefully, let bears know humans are present and should run off to hide.

When in camp, either hang up or place in bear boxes if available, all smellables, including all food, lotions, and insect repellants.

In conclusion, bears are seldom a strong threat on the AT; just leave them alone.

Mice/rodents

Mice and other rodents inhabit just about every shelter and surrounding campground along the AT. Not only are mice and rodents a pain when trying to get to food, but they also have fleas that can carry diseases. When staying at a shelter or campground, expect rodents to take an interest in your food and pack. Many shelters have hanging hooks that have a mouse or rodent deterrent device to protect whatever is hanging from the hook. As I have mentioned before, you should open all pack pockets in case some food crumbs are in the pocket, so a mouse can enter the pocket, eat the crumbs, then exit. Otherwise, the rodent may decide to create an opening into the pocket.

Moose

It's hard to believe how large a moose can be. According to National Park Authorities in Alaska, more people are injured by moose every year than by bears.

When encountering a moose, try not to let it know you are there. If the moose does see you, talk to it in a deep voice and move slowly away. If it charges, you should run and try to get away or get behind something solid, like a tree, boulder, or car. Like bears, moose seldom chase humans. If attacked by a moose, roll up into a ball and try to protect your head with your hands and arms. Lay still until the moose backs away. Unlike black bears, fighting back at a moose only encourages the moose to keep fighting.

NOTE: Moose are seldom a strong threat on the AT if left alone.

Insects

While bears and moose may seem to be the most dangerous threat on the AT, insects are much more likely to cause a severe problem. Mosquitoes can carry diseases, and black flies cause a painful bite that can get infected. Ticks can carry Lyme disease which can cause lifelong debilitation if not caught and treated properly.

The AT goes through an area in New England that must be considered ground zero for Lyme disease. I did whatever I could to prevent contracting this potentially debilitating disease. To mitigate contracting this disease, I took several steps in my hiking preparation as well as during my hikes.

The first step in preventing problems with insects is to avoid them-easier said than done. I started my insect prevention program by purchasing as many of my hiking clothes as possible that had been factory treated with an insecticide called Permethrin.

Permethrin is not an insect repellant but an insecticide that kills insects that come in contact with it. Pyrethrin was developed for our military to treat clothing for our armed forces. By purchasing clothing that had been factory treated, the treatment could take up to 70 washings, or enough to last until the clothing was worn out. I purchased convertible hiking pants with zip-off legs and a hiking shirt from a company called Exo-official that offer treated clothing. I was also able to purchase a buff to wear on my head that was factory treated as well.

The second thing I did was treat my remaining clothing with Permethrin myself. While there are companies that custom treat clothes with Permethrin that will also last through 70 washings, I chose to treat my own.

I did this in two different ways. First, I purchased Permethrin from a farm store, diluted it myself, soaked my clothing in the diluted mixture and allowed the clothing to dry. This method of treating clothing is supposed to be good for at least 7 washings. The second way I treated my clothing was to purchase Pyrethrin on the trail in an already diluted state in a spray bottle and simply sprayed my clothing with it. This method was also supposed to be good for 7 washings. Clothing I treated myself I retreated every few weeks.

The third thing I did to keep from getting Lyme disease was to visit my doctor and get a prescription for an antibiotic called Doxycycline HYC 100MG. This antibiotic is not only used to treat Lyme disease but many different bacterial infections in the body such as urinary tract infections, eye infections, gum disease, and others. My doctor said to take it if I discovered a tick stuck to my body and if I did not know how long it had been on me. He said a tick had to be on a person at least 24 hours before the disease-causing bacteria could be transferred into the body. If I got the tick off in less than 24 hours, I would be fine. If I didn't or did not know for sure, then I was to start taking the drug. He also said if I experienced the signs of Lyme disease starting, then begin treatment immediately with the antibiotic. Signs he said to watch for included a red, "bullseye ring" rash at the site of the bite, muscle and joint pain, headache, chills, fever, swollen lymph nodes, and a general lack of energy.

My doctor had my prescription filled at Walmart, so I would be able to get a refill on the trail if I needed it (but only after calling him). He also warned me to stay out of the sun anytime I was using Doxycycline.

The final thing I did to help protect against Lyme disease was to be extra cautious and keep an eye open for ticks. The ticks that transmit Lyme disease can be extremely small, so this was no easy task, but, fortunately, I never found one on me.

Mosquito bites are another matter as I had exposed skin when hiking the 100-mile wilderness in Maine where mosquitoes are famous for being big, numerous, and hungry! I did have one blackfly bite, and it hurt for a week! To prevent mosquito and other insect bites, I used 100% Deet insect repellent. Some say a lesser concentration of Deet will work, but I figured if I were carrying it, I'd go for the strong stuff! I used a small pump spray bottle when hiking in areas where I needed to use it daily. In areas where I seldom needed insect repellent, I carried a foil pouch with a towelette soaked with Deet. This was lighter and easier to carry as it fit flat inside my first aid pouch.

In summary, there are several steps one can take to avoid insect problems. They include the following:

- Wear treated clothing that is light in color.

- Walk in the middle of the trail, avoid brushing up against bushes, grass, and weeds.

- When sitting down, sit on a pad or ground cloth, especially if it is treated with Permethrin.

- Do a "tick check" nightly and remove ticks with either a pair of tweezers or use a tick key, available at most sporting goods stores or online.

- Camp away from water sources, if possible. Camping on ridges will help keep mosquitoes away.

- Carry the antibiotic Doxycycline if needed to treat Lyme disease.

NOTE: Lyme disease is a REAL threat on the AT, especially in New England.

Porcupines

Many hikers never see a porcupine while hiking on the AT. The biggest threat from porcupines is their quills that can get stuck in the skin and be extremely painful to remove. Most porcupine problems come from dogs on the trail that ended up with a nose full of quills which require the services of a veterinarian.

Poisonous Snakes

Rattlesnakes, Copperheads, and Cottonmouth snakes are the three types of poisonous snakes found along the AT. The best way to handle poisonous snakes is to avoid them by keeping an eye out while hiking. If a poisonous snake is discovered, simply wait till it moves out of the way or walk around it, keeping plenty of room between the snake and you. Never put hands or feet in a place that cannot be seen. Kicking one's feet will let any snake on the trail ahead know something is coming and give it time to move out of the way.

If bitten by a poisonous snake, remain calm and contact 911 immediately. Remove any jewelry or items that could cause problems if swelling should occur. Avoid any strenuous activity. Try to identify the type of snake that inflected the bite or at least note its appearance so medical authorities can determine the correct antivenom to use. Because the AT frequently crosses a road and with many people hiking the trail, getting emergency help should seldom be a problem.

Avoiding Falls

Being an older hiker, I realize that two of the things that made me different from younger hikers were that I could get hurt more easily, and when I did, I would take longer to heal. When I started planning for my first AT hike, I thought that getting hurt was the greatest threat to me completing a thru-hike. I had plenty of time, enough money, the support of my family, and the desire. The one big unknown was my ability to stay healthy, so to avoid falls, I took my time when hiking over roots and rocks. I used trekking poles to give me two additional points of contact with the ground. The only time I never used trekking poles was when I had to use both my hands and feet to navigate up and down rock scrambles.

Avoiding Lower Leg Problems

The major issue long-distance hikers seem to have regarding getting hurt deals with the lower legs. This refers to the knees down. These problems can consist of blisters, Plantar Fasciitis, Peripheral Neuropathy, shin splints, tendonitis, ankle sprains and breaks, stress fractures, general soreness, and swelling. Many long-distance hikers continue to experience lower leg issues long after they complete their hike. These problems usually involve nerve damage that manifests itself as numbness in the toes and the bottoms of the feet but normally heal themselves within a year or so of completing a long distance hike.

As I start this section on how to avoid lower leg problems, I need to say this information was learned the hard way. What caused me to halt my thru-hike and become a section hiker, was not a fall, but from hiking long distances and not knowing how to take care of my feet.

The first lower leg issue I experienced was what most hikers experience first, and that is blisters.

There are two general types of blisters. The first is an abrasion blister where the skin wears away from abrading against something like the inside of a shoe. The fix for this type of blister is simple, put a band-aid over a dab of triple antibiotic on the place that is getting abraded. This way the band-aid takes the punishment and not the skin.

The second type of blister is caused by the outside skin being held in place, but the inside of the foot moving around, causing a fluid buildup underneath the surface of the skin. The treatment for this type of blister is a little more complicated. The fluid must first be drained with a sterilized needle and a bandage put over the blister. After this, a piece of duct tape can be cut the size of the bandage and placed over the bandage. By placing the duct tape over the bandage, the tape is easily removed as needed by simply removing the bandage. The duct tape makes the outside of the bandage slick, so the bandage can slide around which now keeps the movement between the skin and the inside of the foot to a minimum.

After hiking the first 500 miles, my feet hurt so badly I had to leave the trail. The bottoms of my feet had become completely numb, but where my toes attached to my feet were so sore, I could hardly get up off the ground. This was when I had developed Exercise Induced Peripheral Neuropathy or nerve damage in my feet. I also developed numbness in my hands that was also diagnosed as Peripheral Neuropathy. I was able to fix the neuropathy in my hands by switching trekking poles to a brand called PacerPoles. PacerPoles are made in England and have a hand grip offset by 45 degrees that keeps pressure off the wrist and puts it on the side of the hands.

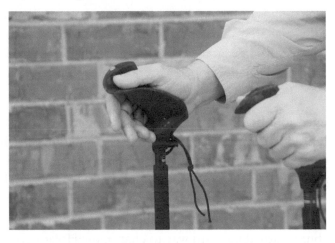

Pacer trekking poles with 45° offset handles

The sad part of this story is I had to hike an additional 1300 miles before I began to understand the cause of, and the ways to prevent, lower leg and foot problems.

The first major thing people can do to avoid lower leg problems is to reduce as much as possible the weight that is felt by the lower legs. This can be done by losing body weight and by reducing the weight carried.

The second major thing people can do to help avoid lower leg problems is to start with hiking short distances and slowly extend the distance hiked. Out of shape hikers should start by hiking from six to eight miles a day and carrying a total pack weight of 15 pounds or less. The distance can slowly be increased provided one does not increase total weekly mileage covered by more than 10% from the previous week.

Taking periodic days off from hiking will also help prevent lower leg problems. I found hiking about six days then taking a Zero-day or a Nero (like a Zero except with a short hike) helped prevent my lower legs from hurting.

Changing brands of hiking shoes went a long way in allowing me to return to the trail after developing Peripheral Neuropathy. In fact, had I understood what was going on with my original hiking shoes, I probably would not have developed as serious neuropathy in the first place.

I changed to a brand of trail running shoe named Hoka. They are generally sold by running stores as well as some outdoor shops. Hoka shoes are known for their lightweight yet highly cushioned sole. I could hardly walk across a hardwood floor barefooted yet could hike the AT wearing these shoes. Because they are so cushioned, they wear out rather quickly. Most shoes should be replaced after hiking 500 miles or so, but I learned the hard way to change my Hoka's every 400 miles. The outside may look fine, but the inside will wear out. Wearing my shoes too long was the major problem that caused me to leave the trail with neuropathy, tendonitis, and finally, plantar fasciitis.

Most shoe companies have liberal return policies that will allow people to use shoes for a while and still take the shoes back. I learned not to hesitate to return shoes that did not feel good on my feet. One final thought about shoe selection: start with buying one size larger than normal. Hikers' feet swell at least this much, so the larger size is needed. After I stopped hiking, my feet took over six months before they would fit into the shoes I had worn before my hikes.

Once shoes have been selected, an upgraded insole for the shoes may be in order. The most popular insoles on the AT appeared to be made by a company named Superfeet. These come in a variety of different heights of arch support. This company also has a liberal return policy so don't hesitate to try various heights of support. When I started to develop Plantar Fasciitis, I started using one size higher up of arch support. This was recommended to me by a doctor in Bangor, Maine, who treated thru-hikers with foot problems. He said this would keep my arch from flexing as much and take pressure off the Plantar Fascia which in turn, would allow it to heal. He also suggested I tape my arch as well to help keep it from flexing. Doing these two things helped me keep hiking.

Socks are the next item for selection. Darn Tough socks are probably the most popular socks on the AT. They come with a lifetime warranty plus they are made in the USA in Vermont. Another brand of sock to consider is Injinji socks. Injinji makes toe socks that many hikers claim to eliminate blisters. These socks come as ultralight weight socks liners or in regular weight to use as hiking socks. I have used both Darn Tough and Injinji sox and got along fine with both brands of socks.

After socks and shoes have been selected, the question arises about using any type of brace on the lower legs. I learned that my knees felt better at the end of a hike if I wore an infrapatellar strap commonly called a Cho Pat strap. These straps are placed under the kneecap and help reduce the strain put on the muscle-tendon that straightens out the leg. I also tried a compression knee sleeve that had copper infused in the sleeve. These worked for me as well as the Cho Pat straps.

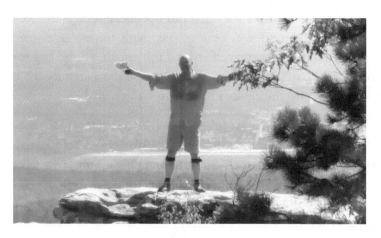

Standing on McAfee Knob with Cho Pat Straps on both knees

Another item to consider using to help prevent lower leg injuries are compression sleeves. These slip up over the foot and compress the lower leg from the ankle to below the knee. I started using these when I developed shin splints by "rock hopping" in Vermont to avoid mud on the trails. A physical therapist I met on the trail told me 80% of the time shin splints are caused by the connecting tissue from the muscle being torn away from the shin bone. He said my leg muscles had strengthened tremendously while hiking the trail, but my connecting tissue was still as weak as it had been when I started. He explained when I started rock hopping, my leg muscles responded with their increased strength that the connecting tissue could not handle. By wearing compression sleeves, some of the stress was taken off the injured connecting tissues, so the pain was reduced. If you look closely at the picture on the cover of this book, you will see my legs are bright pink. I'm not trying to make a fashion statement; I'm simply wearing the only compression sleeves I could find that fit my legs.

Another way to avoid lower leg problems is stretching muscles daily before and after hiking. Having interviewed a sports trainer, along with checking various other sources, it appears all stretching recommendations for hiking involve the muscles from the leg on down, along with the muscles that move the arms. This just about covers any muscle needed to move! Instead of trying to sort through the various stretching exercises, there are enough YouTube videos and websites to allow someone to decide for themselves which ones seem best for their situation.

One product that can help with preventing as well as treating lower leg problems is a product called Kinesiology-Sports Tape or KT Tape. It comes in an assortment of colors and different grades. KT tape is the tape athletes can be seen wearing on their skin. I have seen hikers use it to tape not just knees, ankles, and feet, but arms and elbows as well. Personally, I stick with the highest grade and in precut, 10-inch strips. Once again, there are a plethora of online videos explaining its use. It was KT tape that helped reduce the pain I experienced in my foot when I got Plantar Fasciitis.

Many hikers also use this tape to treat or prevent blisters. The other tape hikers use for this same purpose is called Medical Leukotape Sports Tape. The main difference between KT Tape and Leukotape is KT Tape stretches and can be removed from the skin without much damage. Leukotape, on the other hand, stretches only slightly and removal can be a challenge. I found both to be useful.

Dehydration

Dehydration occurs when a body simply does not have the water it needs. Dehydration can happen because of a variety of reasons such as vomiting, diarrhea, not drinking enough fluids, and sweating. Whatever the cause, dehydration is a serious problem if not treated. The treatment for dehydration is fairly simple provided water, or other liquids are available. Add electrolytes to water, if available.

Heat Exhaustion and Heat Stroke

One would think that a person going by the trail name of Dr. Fix-it, who grew up doing manual labor on a farm in western Kansas, who had been hiking since childhood, who had always enjoyed strenuous activities, who was a certified Wilderness First Aid Responder, would not allow himself to get heat exhaustion. If one believed this, one would be wrong.

It was a sweltering day in early September when I was in Virginia, headed towards Bears Den Hostel. As I hurriedly worked my way over the infamous part of the trail called the *Roller Coaster*, all I could think about was the air-conditioned sleeping quarters at Bears Den, the ice-cold drinks they had in their refrigerator and the Ben and Jerry's Ice Cream they provided to their guests. Before I knew it, I was getting dizzy and lightheaded. Fortunately, I saw a rock beside the trail that was in the shade of a tree. I stumbled over to it and fell on it in a heap. Slowly lowering myself down to the ground, I laid in the shade and started to sip from my water bottle attached to my shoulder strap on my pack. I took the other bottle of water off my other strap and soaked my hat with water and put it back on my head. I then took a small cloth I used to wipe my brow and soaked it with water and placed it on my forehead after I wiped the inside of my wrists with it. Within a few minutes, I could tell my body was responding in a positive way to my heat exhaustion remedies. Obviously, nothing serious became of my stupidity as I am writing about the incident, but the lesson learned has been of utmost importance as I now am much more cognizant of my body and what it is telling me.

Heat exhaustion is when the body generates more heat than it can shed. I had overwhelmed my body's ability to cool itself. I was sweating like crazy which was a good thing. Because I took the actions I did, I was able to avoid the much more serious condition known as heat stroke. Had I stopped sweating, that would be a sign I was having a heat stroke and a very serious medical emergency as fewer than 50% of the victims of heat stroke survive.

The way to avoid heat stroke is to avoid heat exhaustion. The way to avoid heat exhaustion is to drink lots of electrolyte enhanced water or fluids, avoid pushing your body too hard in the hot sun, and to take occasional breaks. It was after this incident that I started to take a lunch break around one in the afternoon. I would find a nice shady spot, eat, then take a nap for about an hour. This delay put me an hour behind for the day, but I simply hiked an hour longer in the cool of the evening which is my favorite time to hike, anyway. I did this until the weather cooled down in the fall.

Hitchhiking

When people hike without their own trail vehicle, they are basically homeless. Being homeless puts folks at the mercy of others when it comes to being transported more than a mile or so. Personally, I prefer to call for a shuttle driver to pick me up instead of taking potluck and seeing if someone will pick up an old man along the road and haul him into town. Shuttle drivers are available almost the entire length of the AT and getting their numbers was seldom a problem. If I did not find a number in a guidebook or from an AT website, I would call a local outfitter, hostel or hotel, or even the local Chamber of Commerce and get the phone number of someone who would give me a lift. I always paid for shuttles, even when people said it was not necessary. I told them this was to encourage them to keep helping hikers.

Only once did I hitchhike. I was with Flash 52. We had taken a taxi into town for the night and had made arrangements to be picked up in the morning. As I awoke the next morning, I got a text from the taxi driver saying her alternate in her car was broken so we would need to find another ride back to the trail. Great. A two-mile hike up a steep hill and we would be ready to start our day on the trail.

We had spent the night at an old resort so as we started to leave, we say a guy through a window, working in the kitchen. We tapped on the window, and he came out. When asked if he knew of anybody who could give us a lift back up the hill to the AT, he pointed across an empty parking lot to a parked car. He said, "See that car? It belongs to Mike. He would be glad to take you back to the trail."

"Where's Mike?" Flash 52 asked. "I'm Mike," was the response.

I would tell the rest of the story, but nobody would believe it. We did, however, get back to the trail in Mike's car. And yes, we were not killed, but we did come close. Never again did Flash 52 and I consider getting a ride from someone other than a taxi company or a shuttle service. However, most AT hikers hitchhike and have no problems.

Hikers who do hitchhike say it is easier for a female to get a ride than a male. Therefore, males should try to get a female to hitch with them.

Hitching from a location where a car can pull over safely and conveniently is also a requirement to hitch a ride easily.

When getting in a vehicle, always hold your pack in your lap if possible. Having a driver drive off with packs in the trunk is rare but possible.

Finally, never get in a vehicle if something does not "feel right." It is always better to be safe than sorry.

Earlier I mentioned I made a sign out of a 20-inch square piece of Tyvek that states "OLD HIKER NEEDS RIDE." While the sign was always available, it provided more laughs on the trail than it was used to hitch a ride. However, many hikers make signs requesting a ride.

Hypothermia

Hypothermia occurs when a body loses more heat than it absorbs or in other words when the core body temperature drops. It can be a real threat on the AT and not just at higher elevations.

Hypothermia can be caused by getting wet with either the wind blowing or during cool temperatures, and not wearing enough clothing for the weather conditions. Mild hypothermia causes a person to start to shiver as the body is trying to generate heat. Mild confusion can occur. The solution is to get dry, get out of the wind and cold, put on more dry clothes, drink hot liquids, and seek out a warm place to allow the body to regain its core temperature by stopping the heat loss that caused the problem in the first place. Severe hypothermia can cause death if not treated promptly.

Illnesses

There are several illnesses to be concerned about when hiking the AT. The most serious are generally insect related, i.e., Lyme Disease transmitted by ticks and diseases caught from mosquitoes such as West Nile Virus and various forms of encephalitis.

The most prevalent illness on the AT is Norovirus, a highly contagious viral infection that is commonly spread through water and food that has become contaminated during preparation or through contaminated surfaces. Norovirus is also contracted through close contact with a person infected with the virus.

Symptoms usually begin from 12 to 48 hours after being exposed to the virus and usually last from one to three days. Symptoms include vomiting, nausea, diarrhea, cramps, fever, and muscle pain. A person can continue to spread the virus through feces for up to two weeks after recovery.

Prevention of Norovirus is the key. This can be done through frequent hand washing with soap along with the use of liquid sanitation products. Hand washing is particularly important after using the bathroom and before eating. The gel type of sanitation products that are most prevalent on the AT, do not help with the prevention of Norovirus. Avoid shaking anyone's hand, but, instead, do a fist or elbow "bump." Many hikers avoid staying in shelters when Norovirus is known to be in the area. It is also good to chemically treat water in addition to filtering it in these areas.

Other illnesses hikers can get are those from tainted water. However, by following proper water treatment procedures, these can be avoided.

Poisonous Plants

The three poisonous plants found along the AT are Poison Ivy, Poison Oak, and Poison Sumac. Poison Ivy and Poison Oak grow as either a bush or a climbing vine. Poison Sumac is either a tree or shrub. While these three plants are not technically poisonous, they do have sticky oil on their leaves called urushiol. Urushiol can cause a blistering, itchy rash after it gets on the skin by simply brushing up against a leaf. The best way to prevent getting this rash is through the avoidance of these plants. When that is not possible, urushiol can be removed from the skin with vigorous washing with soap and water. Once a rash has developed, it can be treated with various over the counter products. More serious rashes are often treated by medical personnel with steroid products.

Staying in Touch

Smart Cell Phones do so much more than just send and receive calls. By utilizing various phone apps, you can use a cell phone to replace both a still and video camera. Also, the smartphone can serve as a GPS to determine location, check distances and elevations to and from various points on or near the trail, check weather and follow storms with radar. By using the camera feature, you can replace the need for copying down information or carrying various books including guidebooks. A smartphone can also have computer file copies of equipment manuals, provide a source for survival information, identify nearby mountain peaks, identify star constellations, receive help and information regarding problems incurred on the trail; the list is practically endless. When relying heavily on a smartphone, carry a backup battery to recharge it in case it becomes discharged before reaching a recharging station. Also, carrying the smartphone in a sealed plastic bag will protect it from moisture from both rain and sweat. If using a trail vehicle, you can have several different sizes of recharging batteries. Select which battery to carry based on the same criteria used to determine how much water or food to carry. It depends upon how far to the next resupply, or in this case, the nest recharge.

The consensus on the AT is that Verizon has the best overall cell phone coverage.

While cell phones give a wonderful way to stay in touch, there are areas along the AT where cell coverage is lacking. If this is a concern, there are two main brands of satellite communicators that can provide contact with the outside world without cell coverage. Both can provide location updates for friends and family to follow your travels. Both also can summon 911 help if needed. The significant differences are in cost and in the ability to customize text messages. Garman Inreach brand is more expensive but does allow for text messages to be sent and received while the other major brand, Spot, does not allow such customization.

Trail Journals are located at all the shelters as well as occasional spots along the trail. They are an additional way of communicating your location with others. By noting when you have been at a shelter, you are not only telling other hikers your general location but in case of emergencies, informing civil authorities of your general location as well.

Stupid light

Andrew Skurka is a well-known and respected ultralight weight trekker. It appears that Andrew coined the term "stupid light" meaning doing stupid things to reduce pack weight. One reason Andrew can safely pack light is that his knowledge of the weather, terrain, his physical abilities, and equipment usage is at a very high level. The question that all ultralight and day hikers must answer is "am I hiking stupid light?" The other question that must always be asked is "Am I underprepared?"

Sunburn

The AT is often called "the green tunnel" because so much of the trail leads through forests. However, in the spring before the leaves come out and in the various sections that are in the open, sunburn is a real possibility. Wearing an appropriate hat to shield off the sun is of great benefit as well as using an appropriate sunscreen lotion on exposed skin. When the leaves come out in the spring, and as you develop a suntan, sunburn becomes less of an issue.

Trailheads/Crazy People

Occasionally people ask if a hiker should carry a gun. The accepted short answer is no. The trail is safe provided one stays situationally aware of what is happening around them. People carrying a pack on the trail are almost always fellow hikers. People without a pack and hanging around a trailhead should probably be viewed as suspicious. The answer here is to avoid staying in shelters close to trailheads (often party spots for locals) and not spending a lot of unnecessary time at trailheads.

During my entire time hiking on the AT, only once did I feel uncomfortable, but I did help other hikers a couple of times. One time I helped a young female hiker by acting like her dad when a few guys were beginning to give her a hard time. Another time I came out to a trailhead and a guy was there with a pickup truck, trying to give a female hiker a ride into town. As I entered the parking area, I heard my fellow hiker say, "Oh, there is my husband now." I at once realized there must be a problem, so I responded by saying, "Sorry I got so far behind. I had trouble with a trekking pole, but I got it fixed." I acknowledged the guy standing by the pickup and then reminded my "wife" we needed to get going if we were going to get our miles in that day so off we headed.

The time I felt uncomfortable was when I was staying at the Doyle Hotel in Duncannon, PA, and I came down to eat dinner in their bar. I noticed a gentleman watching me, and after a while, he got up and weaved his way toward my table. It was obvious he had been in the bar for a bit too long.

He said, "Hey, you must be hiking the trail." I acknowledged the fact he was correct. He then said, "I know who you are." Having been a professional speaker for much of my career, I have met a lot of people over the years who know me, but I do not have a clue who they were, so I asked him how he knew me.

"You are that guy on that TV reality show, Pawn Stars."

"Rick Harrison?" I asked. I figured this because several other people over the years have said I resemble Mr. Harrison.

"Yes, that's who you are, you are Mr. Harrison."

My response was one I was about to regret as I said, "You know people on the AT want to remain anonymous and that is why we go by trail names. I'm Dr. Fix-it."

My answer must have been the wrong answer as my new-found friend was now getting unhappy with me as I would not acknowledge I was Rick Harrison, who he was sure I was. I then had what I consider a stroke of genius, I said, "Hey, how about we take a selfie together? That way you can show people who you met here at the Doyle."

We now became best buds. After taking a couple of selfies together, he weaved back to his table happy as a lark. I wonder what he thought when he woke up the next morning and saw the pictures on his phone.

> *"I know what it is like to be young, but you don't know what it is like to be old."*
>
> **The aging Dr. Fix-it**

Chapter 18

Conclusion

I chose to write this book because I was disappointed in my ability to complete a thru-hike of the AT. I had read many books about how to hike the AT but never found one on how to enjoy it. I now realize the books on how to hike the AT were written by people who are among the 20% of people who were successful in their thru-hike and written for the 20% of people who also will complete their hike. This book is written by a person in the group of 80% who fail for the people who, without this book, would also fail.

The pain I developed in my lower legs kept me from not only loving the experience but would eventually force me to abandon my epic adventure. I don't pretend to be an expert on hiking and backpacking. I did want to simply share some things I would like to have known before I started my hike or at least before I gave up on my original hike. If only I had known then what I know now, perhaps I could have completed my thru-hike.

When I started to determine what was keeping me from being in the 20% of hikers who are successful in their quest, I realized what I was learning would be offensive to some people. I also figured many of those people would be in the group of hikers that were able to complete their hike conventionally. I admire those people that are capable of being in what I call the 20% club. However, when I started my hike, I did not intend to be in the 80% club, and neither did the other members now in this club.

As this book goes to publication, I lack 400 miles to complete my hike of the AT. When I am done, however, my journey will not be over. I intend to keep learning and discovering ways to help others enjoy the outdoors. The last 400 miles on the AT will give me the opportunity to try preparing food using a small gas canister stove as well as trying what is called cold soaking food. To reduce muscle soreness, I will experiment with using a massage stick, massage ball, and a floss band. As far as nutrition, I will be adding a prebiotic to my daily dietary supplement regiment. And finally, I want to try some new products and see if they will be helpful to those who are interested in enjoying the AT.

Once my AT hike is complete, I plan on expanding the KatahdinorBust.com website to include several YouTube videos explaining various equipment modifications and hiking skills in detail. And finally, I hope to keep updating this book with new information that will be helpful to those who don't simply want to hike but want to enjoy hiking as well.

I want to remind everyone that Dana and Jennifer Kee, trail names of Atlas and Matchmaker, were the ones willing to assist this crazy old man in working out the Self Double-Shuttle process. While there were other people who started using the Self Double-Shuttle after we told them what we were doing, I am proud to announce that as far as I know, they were the first to realize their Appalachian Trail Dream, partly because of this process. I hope that they will only be the beginning of the folks who will be able to utilize the information in this book to help fulfill their desired AT experience.

By publishing this book and promoting a new approach to hiking the Appalachian Trail, I will make more friends and more enemies than I have up to this point in my life. I originally wrote this book to be a guide for seniors on how they could enjoy the AT. However, as many young people learned what I was discovering, they adopted many of the techniques I have shared in this book and used them to stay on the trail instead of joining the 80% club.

To my younger critics, I say this: "I know what it is like to be young, but you don't know what it is like to be old." I then add, "My prayer for you is that you are given the opportunity to become my age and if you do, that you are able to come back and relive your AT experience."

As I approach seventy years of age, I am asked by many seniors if they should try to hike the AT. Naturally, I encourage them, but I do have to say this, "Younger would have been easier."

As I conclude this book, let me close with the same words I used to open the introduction.

It had been four days since I had a shower. I stunk so bad the flies started leaving me alone. My muscles hurt in places I did not know I had places. As I continued putting one foot in front of the other, pushing my body over yet another boulder in the trail, I started to cry. I thought, "Man, how can I be so blessed? I'm pushing 70 and hiking the Appalachian Trail."

May God bless you as well.

Gail Hinshaw

aka Dr. Fix-it

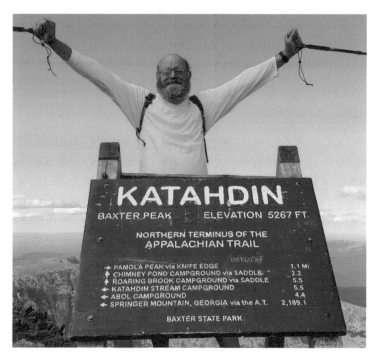

Dr. Fix-it on top of Mt. Katahdin

Appendix

The Story of Flash 52

I met Flash 52 when he walked out of the woods coming down the AT while I was stopped at a stream to filter water. He said, "I finally caught you. I've been following you all day." I told him that nobody follows me, they pass me because I hike slowly to keep from hurting myself. He went on to say he hiked slowly because he was trying to heal his leg from a motorcycle accident and because he could not catch me, nor did I move away, we must hike the same speed. And so, started a friendship that will last a lifetime.

As we started to hike together, the first thing we talked about was gear, as we had packs from the same manufacturer. From there we discover we had the same tent and air mattress! We both had been public speakers, seminar presenters, and business entrepreneurs. He then told me how he got his trail name and about his accident and why he walked with a limp.

He said his trail name was given to him because he hiked slowly. He added the number 52 because there was another Flash on the trail and to distinguish between the two; he added 52 to his name as that was the number of his racing motorcycle. At age 52, he thought it would be fun to get into motorcycle racing. An accident crushed his pelvis into 23 pieces. During surgery, the nerve to his left femur, or thigh bone got pinched, causing him excruciating pain down his leg. At one time, he was on five different pain medications, including the highly addictive Oxycontin.

He continued his story saying one day he told his doctor he could not handle the pain anymore, and his doctor told him he simply was just going to have to learn how to manage his pain. He went home and decided the doctors were unable to help him; he was going to have to take charge of his healing. He started by stopping one of the five pain medicines. When he realized his pain was not any worse with just the four pain medicines, he stopped a second pain medicine. Still, the pain was not any worse. He stopped the third, then fourth, and finally the fifth pain medicine, and still, the pain was not any worse than when he was taking all five medicines.

Flash 52 then told me he announced to his wife he was going to heal himself by going to physical therapy for eight to ten hours a day; he was going to hike the Appalachian Trail. They lived in Maryland, so the trail ran within a couple hours' drive of their home.

Flash 52 had never hiked or backpacked before. However, he did have the internet and YouTube for research and determined what equipment he needed to hike the AT. In 2015, one month before he was planning to start to hike the AT from Springer Mountain, he told his wife he was going to do a four-mile shakedown hike around their neighborhood. A mile from his house, he called home and told his wife come to get him; he could not handle the pain.

Now his story became intriguing when he told me that only one month later, he was at the top of Springer Mountain, ready to hike north. The first day he had to literally drag his body 2 ½ miles to his first camping spot. He continued moving north during 2015 until he had reached Erwin, Tennessee. His total mileage for 2015 was 300 miles.

He picked his hike up in the spring of 2016 at Erwin and continued north.

As we got close to the end of the day, we stopped at a crossroad when he informed me he had a car just down the road at a trailhead parking lot. He asked if I would be interested in going with him to a hostel that night. I said, "You have a car on the Appalachian Trail?"

He answered in the affirmative. I asked again, "You have a car on the Appalachian Trail?"

He once again reassured me that yes, indeed, he had a car. Flash 52 told me he would drive it 40 miles or so up the trail and get a shuttle driver to take him back to where he had gotten off the trail. He would hike a few days to get back to his car at which time he would drive into town, resupply, and go to a hostel to shower and spend the night. He did not use a car the prior year but reported that it helped to have it this year.

He repeated this shuttling maneuver over and over as he made his way north. While I appreciated the offer of a ride and a stay in a hostel, I remembered I had told a couple of other thru-hikers I would meet them at a shelter just a short way up the trail, and if I did not show up, they would worry about me.

"No problem," was Flash 52's response as he said he would drive his car only one day up the trail and leave it at a particular trailhead. He described his car and told me if I wanted to go with him to a hostel the following night, just wait by his car, and he would be day hiking right behind me.

I said, "You can day hike the Appalachian Trail?"

"Yes," he responded. "Some people call it slackpacking." He explained anytime he did not want to carry his heavy pack, he moved his car up the trail just 10 to 12 miles, got a shuttle back to where he got off the trail and hiked back to his car.

The next evening, I came out at the trailhead, and there was a blue Honda Accord with Maryland license plates, just like he said. It appeared to be in decent shape; the tires looked new. I figured I had nothing to lose, so I waited. Flash 52 soon showed up, and we went off to the Rock and Sole Hostel to get cleaned up and have a great dinner. I had stayed at other hostels before, but this one was just special with the hosts, Jody and Craig Stine. (We were honored to get to give Craig his trail name of Ironman because of not only his physical stature but because he showed us a metal statue of an iron man that was located a few miles from their hostel.) Jody fed us like kings, and Craig convinced us we should let him shuttle us for a few days, so we could day hike. We drove Flash's car to our end point for the day, and Craig picked us up there and dropped us off where we had gotten off the trail the night before. We would hike back to Flash's car and then return to the hostel for the night as well as for Jody's cooking for dinner and breakfast. I soon thought to myself, "This is not a bad way to enjoy the AT!"

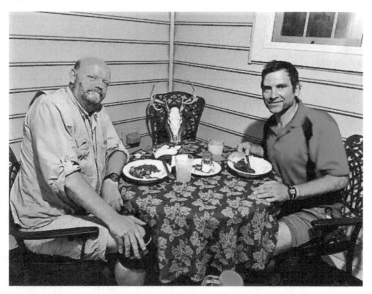

Dr. Fix-it with Flash 52 enjoying dinner at the Rock n' Sole Hostel

For the next 338 miles, it was my privilege to enjoy the AT with Flash 52. Driving his car ahead, shuttling back to the trail and hiking up to the car. Some days we moved the car only one day up the trail, and other days we moved it several days ahead until we reached Dalton, Massachusetts. Flash had to fly to his daughter's wedding, and I went home to nurse my feet back to health as I had developed severe foot problems.

Flash 52 returned to the trail the following week and summited Mount Katahdin on September 25th.

Today his pain is much less, but he is still working daily to completely rid his body of leg pain as well as to walk without a limp.

And now you know why Flash 52 serves as a daily motivator to not only myself, but many others who know his story of grit and determination.

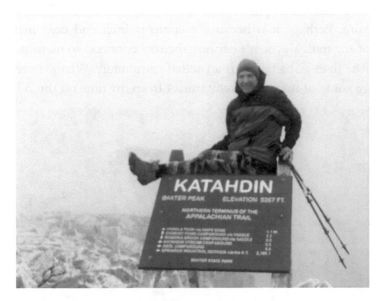

Flash 52 completing his AT hike on Mount Katahdin

The AT is More than a Trail; it's a Community

They call the Appalachian Trail the People's Trail. Why, I'm not quite sure. Perhaps it is because volunteers built and now maintain most of the trail. Maybe it's because the trail connects so many people. It is more than just a trail; it is an actual community. Whatever reason, here are some of my many *people* stories from my time on the AT.

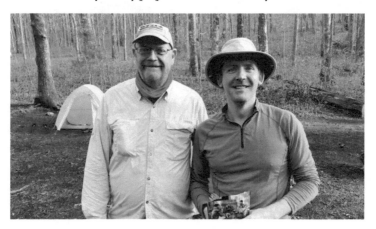

My neighbor's nephew I met on the trail

I met this young man the second night on the trail as I left Springer Mountain. I set up my tent at a campground and saw this young man struggle setting up his tent next to mine. I introduced myself as Dr. Fix-it and asked if I could be of assistance to him in setting up his Six Moons Design tent. He accepted my help, and after studying his tent, we determined if he would lengthen his trekking pole that held up the middle of his tent, then the sides should pull out correctly. He did this, and his tent looked great. He asked where I was from, and I said Branson, Missouri. He said he had spent some time in Branson as he had an aunt and uncle living in the area. Turned out his aunt and uncle not only were my neighbors, but I had been in their home the week just before leaving to hike the trail!

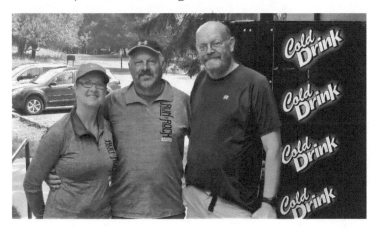

Neighbors of mine from Missouri who shuttled me in Shenandoah National Park

I left my trail vehicle at the north end of Shenandoah National Park and hiked away from it because I could not find a shuttle driver. Knowing the park had one long road through the middle, catching a ride back should be easy as there had to be tourists driving up the length of the park. I was about 70 miles south and figured it was time to go back and get my car. I went to a campground in the park, got a shower, and washed laundry-figuring it would be much easier to get a ride if I did not smell like a hiker. I saw this gentleman sitting by the laundry, so I started talking to him. To make this a short story, ended up, we lived less than 30 miles apart back in Missouri. His wife worked for an organization that was a client of my business. Their daughter had been my grandson's pre-school teacher; their son-in-law was a good friend of a good friend of mine. Their daughter and son-in-law own a body shop that since has fixed my wife's car after she decided to start deer season early with her SUV.

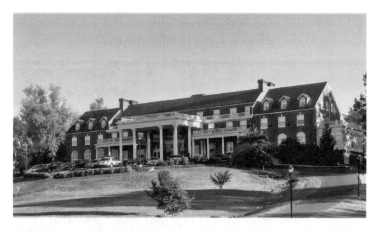

Mimslyn Inn, Luray, Virginia

I drove into Luray, Virginia, planning on taking the next day off the trail to rest and to start writing this book. I went to the Chamber of Commerce building to see where the library was, so I could go there the next day to write and have internet access. The folks there insisted I come back tomorrow and use their conference room to write as it was open until 5:00 PM; plus, I was welcome to use their internet. I asked where a good donut shop was as I loved donuts.

The next morning, I showed up with a dozen donuts. I was treated like a king the entire day. Late in the afternoon, I wrapped up my writing and went out to my vehicle where I called my wife and told her if we ever had to find a new place to live, Luray, Virginia, would have to be at the top of the list. Not only had I been treated well at the Chamber, but I also went to an outfitter in town. Former AT Thru-hiker, Pittsburg, the guy working the store, offered to shuttle me about a hundred miles south and all he wanted was gas money!

As I was getting my hiking stuff ready to go back hiking the next day, a gentleman drove up and introduced himself as Jim Sims. He admired how I was so organized with the chest of drawers in the back of my trail vehicle. He asked if I would like a hotel room for the night as he was the general manager for the Mimslyn Inn. Said he never knew of an AT hiker that would not like a room. Naturally, I took him up.

He said he would call his manager and they would be expecting me. I did not quite know what to expect; it could be a roach hotel as far as I knew. But free is free and free is good.

I could not believe the hotel when I saw it. Turned out to be one of the top historic hotels in America. The doorman greeted me with "Dr. Fix-it, I presume? Right this way." When I got to the front desk, I received the same greeting along with the comment my room was ready. The finest trail magic during my entire AT experience was in Luray, Virginia; a must stop on the AT!

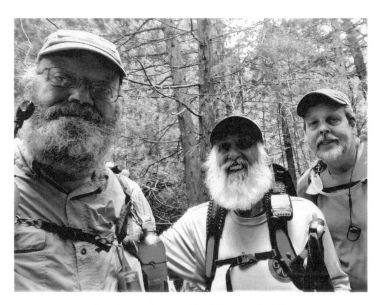

Grey Beard between Dr. Fix-it and Atlas

Atlas and I were hiking south in Maine and saw this gentleman coming toward us (the gentleman in the middle). While we had never met, I knew at once who he had to be. I said to him as he approached, "You must be Grey Beard! We've not met, but I have heard of you." Grey Beard was 82 years young, and if he completed the AT that year, he would be the oldest thru-hiker ever on the AT. We visited for a bit, and I asked him for some advice to share with other seniors about how he was able to carry out such a feat.

He said four things were needed. First, stay active, second, have a spiritual life, third, find your happiness, and finally, eat healthily.

On October 26, 2017, Grey Beard became the oldest person ever to thru-hike the Appalachian Trail.

Ten Steps to Planning Your Hike

1. Start to "affiliate" with the trail by studying the history and current situation of the AT. Read books and hiker blogs, watch movies and YouTube videos.

2. Start telling others of your plans to hike the AT.

3. Select a strategy to enjoy the AT.

4. Create a money budget as well as a time budget. Include a schedule or calendar for our adventure.

5. Visit your family physician to decide if you are physically capable of fulfilling your desired strategy or what you need to do in preparation for your AT adventure. Get proper medications that may be needed to support your AT experience.

6. Figure out if you will be self-shuttling or will you need a support person *back home* that can send you supplies and handle problems as they arise. Even if you self-shuttle, you will probably need someone back home to help with problems that will happen while you are gone.

7. Start selecting equipment needed depending on the strategy you select.

8. Decide transportation to the trail.

9. Start physical preparation for your adventure.

10. Start using your equipment to get comfortable with its use. Consider doing a few "shakedown" hikes to "dial in" your equipment and to help get in physical shape. More day and nights you spend in preparation for your AT adventure, the greater your odds are for your success.

Places to Consider Hiking Along the Appalachian Trail

Originally, I wanted to title this chapter, *Interesting Places to Hike on the Appalachian Trail*. However, what may be interesting to one person may be entirely boring to another. The same thing could be said if I used the title, fun places to hike, easy places to hike or challenging places to hike. Therefore, I chose a title that will allow readers to investigate the places and decide for themselves if these are locations they might want to hike. Here are my suggestions for portions of the AT one should consider and look forward to hiking.

Georgia

Georgia is the home of the southern end of the AT. Therefore, the southern terminus of the AT is one place to consider visiting. Go to Amicalola Falls State Park and check out the visitors' center where hikers check-in. There is a gift shop with plenty of AT paraphernalia for sale. Watch hikers weigh their packs on the scales on the porch. Walk out the back of the visitors' center, under the arch over the trail that leads to Amicalola Falls and hike to see the falls.

Ask for a road map and directions to get to the forest road that leads to the top of Springer Mountain. The forest road is a dirt road but easily drivable in a car. There is a large parking lot where the AT crosses the road. Hike the one mile to the top of Springer Mountain to see the plaque marking the south end of the trail. Read some entries in the trail journal stored at the base of the marker. See the southernmost AT trail blaze before hiking back to the car.

A three day, 31-mile hike from the southern end of the trail to Neel Gap at US 19 gives a feel for the AT. This stretch of trail causes up to 25% of the potential thru-hikers to quit. Most all the hikers on this part of the trail in the spring will be northbound newbies, trying to figure out their equipment as well as what they are doing. In the fall of the year, some of the hikers will be southbound thru-hikers completing their journey. Arriving at Neel Gap in the spring is an experience as there is both an outfitter and a hostel at this major road junction. Most hikers resupply here or catch a ride into a nearby town to resupply. It is quite a circus with so many hikers calling it quits and those that are reconsidering their equipment choices. The hikers that stay on the trail mail home an average of four and a half pounds of equipment.

North Carolina

The Great Smoky Mountains National Park is a wonderful place to hike. The AT goes from Fontana Dam, 164 miles from Springer Mountain, up to the ridge of the Smoky Mountains to Clingman's Dome which is 199 miles from Springer. It is also the highest point on the entire AT. There is a parking lot with road access to Newfound Gap, US Highway 441, which crosses the AT five miles further up the trail. US Highway 441 runs from Gatlinburg, TN to Cherokee, NC, both places interesting to visit. The AT then continues through Smokey Mountain National Park for an additional 30 miles to Davenport Gap where it crosses highway TN 32 or NC 284. The AT follows the state line between North Carolina and Tennessee throughout the park.

Another fabulous place to see is Max Patch Bald, 253 miles from Springer. It is less than a two-mile round-trip hike from NC SR 1182 parking lot. This wide-open mountaintop offers a fantastic view of Mount Mitchell to the east and equally magnificent views of the Great Smoky Mountains to the west. This place is a short drive from Hot Springs, North Carolina, which has naturally occurring hot springs, a wonderful place to relieve the stress from hiking!

Max Patch Bald is also only 15 miles north of the north end of the Smoky Mountains National Park.

Tennessee

The AT goes through the Smoky Mountains National Park which is on the North Carolina and Tennessee border. Any hike within the park will be on well-maintained trails.

Tennessee is home to Erwin, the only town known to have hung an elephant-interesting but sad event. Erwin is a great AT trail town with lots of support services for hikers.

The hike from Carvers Gap, Tennessee Highway 143, and North Carolina Highway 261, to US highway 19 goes over several balds or bare-topped mountains with views in every direction. Carvers Gap is 379 miles from Springer. This 15-mile hike is especially beautiful if the weather is sunny. In severe weather, this hike would not be so great.

Virginia

Virginia has one-fourth of the entire AT within its borders, so naturally, there are many interesting places to see. Starting at the south end of the trail in Virginia is Damascus, home to the annual AT Trail Days reunion event. Damascus is 469 miles from the south end of the AT. Twenty thousand hikers, former hikers, as well as AT lovers in general, gather here the first weekend after Mother's Day every year. Many vendors are present, selling their wares, repairing hikers' gear, and visiting with customers in general. This is a must-attend event at least once for anybody who loves the AT.

Just a few miles north of Damascus, the AT enters the Grayson Highlands State Park, home to dozens of wild ponies. This is a very popular section of the trail, and when you see this section, you will understand why so many people hike this park. The diversity of trail experiences in this section is amazing. The trail goes over mountain balds, through both hardwood and pine forests, across beautiful meadows, has some rock scrambles, a gorgeous patch of rhododendrons, and it has the wild ponies! Start hiking at Virginia Highway 600 at Elk Garden (493 miles from Springer Mountain) and head north. The first place with a trailhead is in eight miles at Massie Gap with a trailhead two-tenths of a mile east of the trail. The next viable trailhead is at Fox Creek, Virginia Highway 603, another ten miles to the north.

Virginia promotes what is referred to as the "Triple-Crown" on the AT. This is made up of the Dragon's Tooth rock monolith at mile 700 from Springer, McAfee Knob is twelve miles further up the trail at mile 712 from Springer, and finally, at mile 717.6 from Springer, you will find Tinker Cliffs, a half mile cliff walk that looks back to McAfee Knob. There are several access points along the AT shown in the guidebooks.

Another great place to hike the AT is a one hundred mile stretch of trail in the Shenandoah National Park. The trails are well maintained, and food availability is outstanding. There are not many elevation changes throughout the park. Plus, road access is in abundance with the trail constantly crossing over and back the Blue Ridge Parkway that runs alongside the entire length of the park. The views looking out over the countryside are all along the trail.

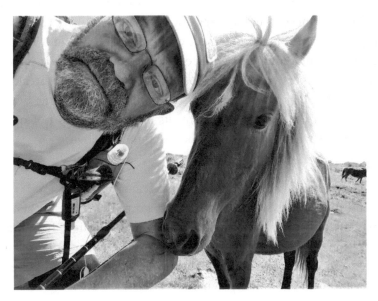

Selfie with one of the ponies in Grayson Highlands State Park

West Virginia

West Virginia is home to just a few miles of the AT. Most notable place on the AT within West Virginia is the town of Harpers Ferry, 1,023 miles from Springer. Not only is Harpers Ferry a very historical place with many downtown buildings of historical note, but it is also

GAIL HINSHAW

home to the Appalachian Trail Conservancy. All thru-hikers need to stop by the office, get their picture taken, and their hiking progress noted. Harpers Ferry is considered the "psychological midpoint" on the AT. The actual midpoint is a few miles further north, just west of Pine Grove Furnace State Park, Pennsylvania.

Maryland

Maryland has 40 miles of some of the easiest hiking on the AT. The area is also home to many Revolutionary and Civil War history. The trail goes by the first monument made to honor George Washington. It also crosses the historic *national road*, dating back to the founding of our country. This crossing is at Turner's Gap, US Alternate 40, 1,041 miles from the south end of the AT. Located at the junction of this road and the AT is the Old South Mountain Inn, probably the finest restaurant actually on the AT. Hikers can camp at nearby Dahlgren AT campground, clean up in the free showers, then have an elegant dining experience. The restaurant is not open for breakfast, so hikers will want to select a take-out dish for breakfast. I chose Key-Lime pie! It did taste good the following morning, but after being hung in a bear bag overnight, its appearance was not quite as spectacular as when served from the restaurant kitchen.

Pennsylvania

Pennsylvania is often called Rocksylvania and for a good reason. It is said this state is where hiking shoes go to die. The southern end of the state is fine with wonderful hiking through breathtaking countryside's. However, once the AT leaves the sleepy little trail town of Duncannon, the rocks attack with a vengeance. The good news is the elevation change is fairly benign.

One famous place on the AT that has attracted hikers for years is the Doyle Hotel. At least stop by and have a meal in the bar. One can also stay a night or two for additional stories to tell.

New Jersey

Southern New Jersey starts like Pennsylvania ends-with rocks. The good news is once you get past the first 30 miles heading north, the rocks dissipate, and the trail becomes more enjoyable.

The first glacial pond on the AT, when hiking from the south, is Sunfish Pond at 1300 miles from Springer. Because this is the first glacial pond northbound thru-hikers see, it appears quite beautiful, which it is. However, this is only the first of dozens of ponds that are all breathtaking. Continuing on north an additional four miles leads to the AMC Mohican Outdoor Center, a must stop. It has a limited food resupply, a food grill, and a quiet library-like setting allowing hikers to simply relax and read a book from their large selection. This is a great place to stop and spend a day.

New York

New York has many interesting places on the AT. The New York City skyline is visible from a couple of locations on the trail, provided the weather is clear. The lowest elevation point on the AT is in a zoo at the base of Bear Mountain, 1,403 miles north of Springer Mountain. The trail goes right through the zoo (free to thru-hikers) then crosses the Hudson River before going up a steep mile climb to a half mile side trail that leads to a rock formation called Anthony's Nose. The view is spectacular from here, looking back on the Hudson River Valley over to the New York skyline.

Connecticut

The AT across Connecticut is all nice hiking. However, the section from Bull's Bridge Road just south of the New York/Connecticut line at 1,460 miles from Springer to the road leading into the town of Kent, CT Highway 341, provides seven and a half miles of very enjoyable hiking. It does cross the New York border twice and goes over Schaghticoke Mountain.

Massachusetts

The trail starting at Webster Road at mile 1,543 from Springer and all the way to Dalton at mile 1,569 is nothing but pure pleasure. Level but with plenty of forests, the highlight is Upper Goose Pond Shelter. It is a wonderful retreat to spend a night but bring your sleeping bag as the bunks are padded. However, no bedding is provided. A pancake breakfast is offered but expect to help with its preparation. There are also canoes available to go paddling on a beautiful pond

Mount Greylock at the north end of the AT in Massachusetts has at its summit, a nice lodge with a fine restaurant. There is also a very inspiring war memorial. One can drive up to the summit or hike up from Cheshire. Just below the summit on the Cheshire side of the AT, is a mountain pond with a small cabin right at the water's edge. It is as pretty as any pond on the entire AT. Only the ponds in Maine equal it in beauty.

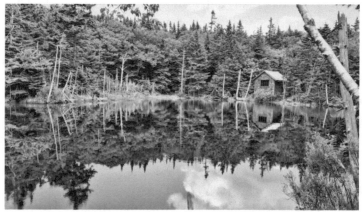

Pond on Greylock Mountain, just below the summit

Vermont

The mountains in Vermont are called the Green Mountains for a reason. The last 45 miles of the AT in Vermont when hiking north, runs through a dense and beautiful forest. Any of this stretch of trail is well worth considering. Vermont is home to the Long Trail which is the same trail as the AT for about half the way across Vermont before it splits off and heads to the Canadian border. Manchester Center is home to the Green Mountain House Hostel, a fabulous place to stay, whether you are hiking the AT or the Long Trail.

New Hampshire

New Hampshire, along with Maine, is home to some of the most difficult areas to hike on the AT, but, it also promises some of the most beautiful sights on the AT. Most hikers say when going through the White Mountains, they could only cover half the normal distance each day they had been covering because of the strenuous nature of the trail. The White Mountains are also subject to some of the absolute worst weather to be experienced on the AT. Add to this the fact that there are miles of exposed trail above timberline, and with the possibility of rapidly changing weather, hiking this part of the AT is only for the well prepared. The Appalachian Mountain Club maintains a series of huts that provide not only shelter but meals as well. While the price to stay at the huts may seem high to most hikers, the huts do fill up. If planning on staying at any of the huts, reservations are recommended. Mount Washington is by far the most famous mountain peak in New Hampshire as well as the most accessible with not only hiking trails to the summit, but a road and cog railroad as well. The top of Mount Washington can become a zoo on beautiful days, especially on weekends. There is a reason for this, and that is the views are spectacular! No matter how one gets to the top of Mount Washington, it must be experienced.

Maine

Southern Maine hosts what many consider the most challenging, as well as the most fun, mile to hike on the entire AT. This mile is called the Mahoosuc Notch, 1,915 miles north of Springer Mountain. This notch has had house-sized boulders tumble down the mountainsides and fill the bottom of the notch. The AT runs right over, as well as through, these boulders. Most hikers plan on up to four hours to crawl, climb, and otherwise navigate through this boulder pile.

After a series of mountains, the AT enters the 100-mile wilderness, 2,075 miles from the south end of the AT. There are several roads with parking at trailheads that access the AT during this 100-mile wilderness. However, the roads are private, and one must pay to drive on them. There is one other item that makes this area a wilderness. No food stops are along this part of the trail. However, food drops are available from Shaw's Hostel in Monson, Maine, along with the White House Landing Camps, a hunting camp that will accept packages for hikers. By utilizing these two services, no more than three days of food would need to be carried. Shaw's in Monson also offers shuttle services along with The Appalachian Trail Lodge, a hostel in Millinocket, Maine. Between the two hostels, it's possible to day hike all across the 100-mile wilderness. Stopping at Shaw's Hostel in Monson is a requirement to appreciate the AT experience to the fullest for several reasons. First, hikers are about to enter the 100-mile wilderness, so Shaw's allows hikers one last place to prepare for this section of the trail. Second, up to the minute information about the upcoming trail is available. And Third, the breakfast at Shaw's is fantastic. The only breakfast I found better on the AT was at Mountain Harbor Hostel, Roan Mountain, Tennessee.

The last 50 miles right before arriving at Mount Katahdin is as level as any part of the trail since Pennsylvania. There are many tree roots, but the trail has little elevation change.

Finally, Maine has beautiful Mount Katahdin in Baxter State Park. The trails to the top of Mount Katahdin are so popular, there are several restrictions on when one can hike to the top. If possible, summit Katahdin on a sunny day. The views are simply indescribable, and the feeling of accomplishment is overwhelming.

Outstanding Hotels and Hostels Along the Appalachian Trail

This list of hotels and hostels is provided to give a perspective of the number of outstanding housing accommodations along the Appalachian Trail. While I have been to most of them, there are a few that I missed, but their reputation among AT hikers is good. For updated contact information, that can change from year to year, please check the various guidebooks as well as online. Almost all either offer shuttles to and from the trail or know people who do.

Georgia
Len Foote Hiker Inn
706-429-0224
Dawsonville, GA

Barefoot Hills Hotel (Formerly Hiker Hostel)
470 788-8044
Dahlonega, GA

Mountain Crossings
706 745-6095
Blairsville, GA

Top of Georgia Hostel and Hiking Center
706 982-3252
Hiawassee, GA

North Carolina
Baltimore Jack's Place Hostel
828 524-4403
Franklin, NC

Gooder Grove Adventure Hostel
828 332-0228
Franklin, NC

Budget Inn of Franklin
828 524-4403
Franklin, MC

Nantahala Mountain Lodge
828 321-2340
Aquone, NC

Cabin in the Woods
828 735-3368
Stecoah Gap, NC

Elmer's Sunnybank Inn
828 622-7206
Hot Springs, NC

Hostel at Laughing Heart Lodge
828 622-0165
Hot Springs, NC

Greasy Creek Friendly
828 688-9948
Bakersville, NC

Harmony Hostel
828 898-6200
Banner Elk, NC

Tennessee

Standing Bear Farm
423 487-0014
Hartford, TN

Hemlock Hollow Inn
423 787-1736
Greeneville, TN

Uncle Johnny's Nolichucky Hostel
423 735-0548
Erwin, TN

Cantarroso Farm
423 833-7514
Erwin, TN

Mountain Harbor B&B and Hiker Hostel
423 772-9494
Roan Mountain, TN

Vango & Abby Memorial Hostel
423-772-3450
Roan Mtn, TN

Doe River Hiker Rest
575 694-0734
Roan Mountain, TN

Kincora Hiking Hostel
423 725-4409
Hampton, TN

Black Bear Resort
423 725-5988
Hampton, TN

Boots Off Hostel and Campground
239 218-3904
Hampton, TN

Virginia

Damascus Old Mill Inn
276 475-3745
Damascus, VA

Dave's Place
276 475-5416
Damascus, VA

Crazy Larry's
276 475-7130
Damascus, VA

The Place
276 475-3441
Damascus, VA

Woodchuck Hostel
406 407-1272
Damascus, VA

Broken Fiddle Hostel
276 608-6220
Damascus, VA

Hikers Inn
276 475-3788
Damascus, VA

Sufi Lodge B&B and Hiker Hostel
276 677-0195
Troutdale, VA

Relax Inn
276 783-5811
Rural Retreat, VA

Quarter Way Inn
276 522-4603
Ceres, VA

Appalachian Dreamer Hiker Hostel
276 682-4061
Ceres, VA

Woods Hole Hostel
540 921 3444
Pearisburg, VA

Angel's Rest Hiker Haven
540 767-4076
Pearisburg, VA

MacArthur Inn
540 726-7510
Narrow, VA

Four Pines Hostel
540 309-8615
Catawba, VA

Stanimal's 328 Hostel
540 290-4002
Waynesboro, VA

Grace Hiker Hostel
540 949-6171
Waynesboro, VA

Mimslyn Inn
540 743-5101
Luray, VA

Open Arms
540 244-5652
Luray, VA

Mountain Home Bed and Breakfast
540 692-6198
Royal, VA

Bears Den Hostel
540-554-8708
Bluemont, VA

Blackburn AT Center
540 338-9028
Round Hill, VA

West Virginia
Teahorse Hostel
304 535-6848
Harpers Ferry, WV

Maryland
Harpers Ferry Hostel
301 834-7652
Knoxville, MD

Pennsylvania
Trail of Hope Hostel
717 360-1481
East Fayetteville, PA

Ironmaster's Mansion Hostel
717 486-410
Gardners, PA

Allenberry Resort
717 258-3211
Boiling Spring, PA

The Doyle Hotel
717 834-6789
Duncannon, PA

Rock N' Sole Hostel
570 617-6432
Summit Station, PA

Blue Mountain Summit
570-386-2003
Andreas, PA

Church of the Mountain Hiker Center
570 476-0345
Delaware Water Gap, PA

New Jersey
Mohican Outdoor Center
908 362-5670
Blairstown, NJ

New York
Anton's on the Lake
845 477-0010
Greenwood Lake, NY

Stony Point Center
845 786-5674 Ext. 100
Fort Montgomery, NY

Connecticut
Bearded Woods Bunk and Dine
860 480-2966
Sharon, CT

Maria McCabe's House
860 435-9577
Salisbury, CT

Vanessa Breton's House
860 435-9577
Salisbury, CT

Massachusetts
Jess' Place
860 248-5710
Sheffield, MA

Vermont
Green Mountain House
330 388-6478
Manchester Center, VT

Hiker Hostel at the Yellow Deli
802 683-9378
Rutland, VT

New Hampshire
Tigger's Tree House
603 643-9213
Hanover NH

Hikers Welcome Hostel
603 989-0040
Glencliff, NH

The Notch Hostel
603 348-1483
North Woodstock, NH

Hiker's Paradise at Colonial Fort Inn
603 466-2732
Gorham, NH

White Mountain Lodge and Hostel
603 466-5049
Shelburne, NH

White Birches
603-466-2022
Shelburne, NH

Maine

Pine Ellis Lodging
207 392-4161
Andover, ME

The Cabin
207 362-1333
Andover, ME

The Hiker Hut
207 897-8984
Rangeley, ME

Farmhouse Inn
207 864-3113
Rangeley, ME

The Rangely Inn
207-864-3341
Rangeley, ME

Stratton Motel
207 246-4171
Stratton, ME

Sterling Inn
207 672-3333
Caratunk, ME

The Caratunk House
207 672-434
Caratunk, ME

Shaw's Hiker Hostel
207 997-359
Monson, ME

White House Landing
207 745-5116
Millinocket, ME

Appalachian Trail Lodge
207 723-4321
Millinocket, ME

Outstanding Companies

The following companies, in my opinion, all make quality products and provide outstanding customer service. The first list consists of companies that I personally enjoy using their products or services.

The second list is comprised of companies that make and distribute lightweight and ultralightweight equipment of interest to hikers and backpackers. Most are considered "cottage" industries based in the United States. Many do custom work as many of their items are made to order. All have a good reputation from AT hikers.

My Favorite Manufacturers

- Enlightened Equipment *www.enlightenedequipment.com*
  Enlightened Equipment makes great sleeping bags and quilts at a fair price. I have never heard anything bad about their products.

- Hoka Hiking Shoes *www.hokaoneone.com*
  Hoka shoes are known as the shoe to wear if foot pain develops. They are lightweight yet highly cushioned. They have a great return policy to ensure their customers get the right shoe. The downside is because of the cushioning in their shoes; their shoes wear out more quickly than most other shoes. I only get 350 to 400 miles before the cushion is gone. However, these shoes will allow me to hike the AT when I have so much foot pain I cannot walk barefoot across a hardwood floor.

- Pacer Poles *www.pacerpole.com*

  Based in England, PacerPole manufactures a revolutionary style of trekking pole with a 45° offset handle that relieves the pressure put on the wrists when hiking and puts the pressure on the side of the hand where it feels much more comfortable. Their website has great videos explaining how the offset handles work. These poles relieved the numbness and nerve damage in my hands.

- Z-packs *www.zpack.com*

Z-packs is a company that is owned and operated by people who take hiking and backpacking seriously. They are on the cutting edge when it comes to ultralightweight equipment and manufacture a wide variety of shelters, backpacks, sleep systems, and a variety of hiking accessories. Until they prove me wrong, I trust anything they sell.

My Favorite Distributors

- Amazon *www.amazon.com*
Amazon gets mentioned as a supplier many hikers come to depend on throughout their hike. The only problem I experienced with Amazon was trying to get an order shipped to general delivery to a United States Post Office. I learned always to have items shipped to a business, so I did not have to plan on being at a Post Office during business hours.

- Recreational Equipment, Inc. (REI) *www.rei.com*
REI is a juggernaut in the world of outdoor sports equipment distribution. As a cooperative, customers have the opportunity to buy a lifetime membership that entitles them to receive a store credit of 10% on all their purchases back at the end of the year. I have been a member since 1968 with a membership number so low, when I go to check out, many store associates get the manager to come over and visit with me. REI has a very knowledgeable and helpful staff. Also, they have a one year, no questions asked, return policy. The only downside to REI is a liberal return policy requires them to sell equipment that is bulletproof. Bulletproof means it is well made from heavy duty materials but leaves much of the ultralightweight equipment to be made and sold by companies like Z-packs. However, REI still offers equipment that approaches the weight of equipment offered by the ultralightweight equipment companies.

I believe that the only reason Walt Disney could call Disneyland the *Happiest Place on Earth* was that he never went to an REI store.

- Bass Pro Shop *www.basspro.com and www.cabelas.com*
  Bass Pro Shop and their sister company, Cabelas, both cater to outdoor sports people in general. Hiking and backpacking are not their specialties, but they do offer a broad selection of equipment, clothing, and hiking shoes. One of the things I like most about these companies is their owner is dedicated to not just preserving the great outdoors but helping people get out and enjoy it as well.

Makers and sellers of lightweight and ultralightweight equipment of interest to hikers and backpackers

- AntiGravityGear *www.antigravitygear.com*
  Shelters, accessories, and more

- Bear Paw Wilderness Designs *www.bearpawwd.com*
  Lightweight shelters and accessories

- Big Sky International *www.bigskyinternational.com*
  Freestanding shelters

- DIY Gear Supply *www.diygearsupply.com*
  Materials, fabrics, hardware and just about anything else needed to build DIY gear

- Elemental Horizons *www.elementalhorizons.com*
  Backpacks and accessories

- Equinox LTD *www.equinoxltd.com*
  Backpacks, shelters, accessories and more

- Feathered Friends *www.featheredfriends.com*
  Down sleeping bags and clothing

- Gossamer Gear *www.gossamergear.com*
  Backpacks, shelters, sleep systems & more

- Hammock Gear *www.hammockgear.com*
  Hammock tarps, quilts, and accessories

- Hennessy Hammock *www.hennessyhammock.com*
  Hammock shelters

- Hyperlite Mountain Gear *www.hyperlitemountaingear.com*
  Dyneema fiber backpacks, shelters, and accessories

- Integral Designs *www.integraldesigns.com*
  Shelters, bivys and accessories

- Jacks R Better *www.jacksrbetter.com*
  Sleeping quilts, shelters, and accessories

- Katabatic Gear *www.katabaticgear.com*
  Sleeping quits and bivys

- LightHeart Gear *www.lightheartgear.com*
  Double-wall shelters, fabrics, and accessories

- LW Gear *www.lwgear.com*
  Backpacks, DVDs, books, and videos

- Nunatak *www.nunatakusa.com*
  Sleeping quilts and down apparel

- Mountain Laurel Designs *www.mountainlaureldesigns.com*
  Backpacks, shelters, sleep systems and more

- Outdoor Equipment Supplier LLC
  www.outdoorequipmentsupplier.com
  Tarps, shelters, and accessories

- Outdoor Vitals Live Ultralight *www.outdoorvitals.com*
  Inexpensive sleep systems, and accessories

- Oware *www.owareusa.com*
  Shelters, sleep systems, and accessories

- Six Moons Designs *www.sixmoondesigns.com*
  Backpacks, shelters, and accessories

- Suluk 46 *www.suluk46.com*
  Backpacking tools and accessories

- Tarptent *www.tarptent.com*
  Single and double-wall shelters

- Trail Designs *www.traildesigns.com*
  Stoves, cookware, and accessories

- Ultralight Adventure Equipment *www.ula-equipment.com*
  Backpacks

- Western Mountaineering *www.westernmountaineering.com*
  Down sleeping bags and apparel

Resources

There are numerous resources to assist in planning and executing your enjoyment of the AT. Most applications are available for various smartphone operating systems. There are many other smartphone applications not listed here regarding the AT, and more are being added all the time. Be sure to search your smartphone's application store for the latest ones.

Books

Numerous E-books are available in the various E-Book formats or as PDF files.

- *AWOL on the Appalachian Trail* by David Miller

  David Miller has written a great narrative of his 2003 through hike. This book lets you know what to expect before you get there. David has been publishing The A.T Guide every year. See below.

- *The A.T. Guide by* David "Awol" Miller

  This book has two editions every year, Northbound and Southbound. The information is the same except the layout is either in the Northbound direction or Southbound direction. The A.T Guide by AWOL is recommended to be downloaded as a PDF file as the trailheads have GPS Coordinates that makes it extremely easy to locate them on Google or Apple Maps. Having the GPS coordinates makes it easy to drive to the trailheads.

- *The Don's Bother Method; How I thru-Hiked the Appalachian Trail and Rarely Slept in the Woods* by Mike Stephens

  This book goes into depth on how Mike Stephens slackpacked the AT. Stephens shares the locations of each night's stay, the distance hiked each day, and other valuable information for anyone contemplating day hiking the AT.

- *The Slack Packers Guide to Hiking the Appalachian Trail* by Lelia Vann and Greg Reck

This book details how this husband and wife team thru-hiked the AT by slackpacking most of the way. Between this book and Mike Stephens' book, readers will get to understand the logistics of using outside shuttle services to assist in day hiking the AT.

- *Thru-Hikers' Companion Guide* by Appalachian Trail Conservancy

This book has similar information at The A.T. Guide but in slightly different format. I had both books downloaded on my smartphone so that I would have the advantage of two sources of information. This book is published yearly.

- *Ultralight Backpackin' Tips* by Mike Clelland

This book is a great source of information regarding how to lighten your pack.

- *Walkin' with the Ghost Whisperers, Traditions and Lore of the Appalachian Trail* by J.R. "Model-T" Tate

J.R. "Motel-T" Tate shares many stories about areas and things found along the trail. This book is interesting reading before hiking through an area. There were times I would come upon something unusual, such as a large mound of rocks that were stacked up on top of a mountain. I would want to know, why? This book explains some of these unusual sightings as well as the history of various areas along the trail.

Internet Websites

Many websites on the internet are helpful for learning about and planning an Appalachian Trail experience.

- *Appalachiantrail.org*

  This website is probably the first place to start planning your AT experience. This website is run by the Appalachian Trail Conservatory and has much information of interest for AT hikers.

- *Sectionhiker.com*

  A great website for beginners as well as experienced backpackers to gain knowledge about hiking and backpacking in general.

- *Thetrek.co*

  The Trek is another outstanding website with lots of articles, blogs, and discussion forums to help plan a long-distance hike.

- *Trailjournals.com*

  This website is home to many hikers who are posting their trail journals. It is informative to follow people who are ahead of you on the trail, so you will know what is coming up. Also, it is fun to simply pick a couple of hikers and follow them on their journey and live vicariously through them.

- *YouTube.com*

  YouTube has many videos made by AT hikers and backpacking enthusiasts. The best advice I can give is simply to do some searches and discover those that appear to meet your information needs. Avoid gear list videos of people before they hike the A.T. Many don't know any more than you. Watch the gear lists of people after they have completed the trail.

The three YouTube channels I have learned the most from are "Follow Bigfoot," "Darwin onthetrail" and Dixie at her channel "Homemade Wanderlust." These people are doing the outdoor community a great service by providing great information based on their real-world experience.

- *Warrendoyle.com*

Warrendoyle.com is the website to Dr. Warren Doyle, a retired college professor who has traversed the AT a total of 17 times, more than any other person. (That is 36,000 miles!) Dr. Doyle has different training programs available that have proven to increase a person's chance of being successful thru-hiking the AT.

- *WhiteBlaze.net*

WhiteBlaze is both a smartphone application and website. It is a discussion forum to help answer questions about hiking the AT.

SmartPhone Applications

- *Amazon Kindle*

Various E-books are available in this format that could prove both interesting as well as helpful. See the section on recommended books.

- *Appalachian Trail Weather*

Mile markers drive this weather application. Type in the appropriate mile marker on the trail and several shelters will pop up both behind and ahead of the mile marker. The weather forecast for the next week will be displayed for several shelters around the mile marker selected.

- *Guthook's AT Guide*

While there are several GPS apps available, the most popular at the time of this writing is called *Guthook's AT Guide*. It not only gives maps of the entire trail, but shows the current location of the hiker. It also shows distances to and locations of shelters, water sources, trailheads, points of interest, as well as a wealth of general information important to hikers, in general; this application is **a must-have for AT hikers**.

- *MyRadar*

This app provides up to the minute weather radar that shows the location of the user in relation to the current weather.

- *Peak Visor*

This app will identify mountain peaks by simply pointing a phone at a mountain range. The cost is around $5.00.

- *SkyView Free*

For those into stargazing, you might want to consider this free smartphone application. Simply point your phone to the sky, and it will identify various celestial objects.

- *WhiteBlaze* and *WhiteBlaze.net*

WhiteBlaze is both a smartphone application and website. It is a discussion forum to help answer questions about hiking the AT.

- *Youtube and Youtube.com*

Youtube is a fantastic way to not only share your video's to your friends and family, but it is also a great way to study and learn about the trail, equipment, food, and just about anything else related to just about anything. There are three people, in particular, to follow on YouTube. They are *Follow Bigfoot*, *Darwin Onthetrail*, and Dixie on her Youtube channel, *Homemade Wanderlust*.

Gear List and Revisions

The following pages show the equipment I carried and how it changed during my hikes on the AT. Hopefully, careful study will reveal the change in philosophy and the reduction in fears I had from the time I started my AT hikes.

The first column lists the items and their weight I started with on my planned thru-hike. The second column shows the items and their weights when I returned to the trail as a section hiker, having had to stop my thru-hike.

The third column illustrates my gear list and weights when I returned in the spring of 2017 to complete my AT hike. The final column displays my day hiking gear.

At the bottom of the lists are four different total weights shown. The first weight shown is pack base weight or the weight of only those items carried with the pack and are not consumed while on the trail.

The second weight shown is the pack base weight plus the weight of the items consumed on the trail. Major consumables are food and water. Other consumables are fuel for cooking and toilet paper. There were days ibuprofen could have been included.

The third weight shown is the weight of the items I carried on my body such as clothes, cell phone, glasses, and anything else I had in my pockets.

The final weight shown is called "skin out" weight, meaning the weight of everything carried from the skin out.

There is one other weight nobody seems to talk about, and that is what I call "knee weight." This is the total weight that must be supported by one's knees. It is this weight that the lower legs must contend with every step and may be the most important weight of all. Naturally, one's body type will help determine if body weight is good or bad. Males tend to lose body weight while doing long distance hikes while females tend not to lose weight. Everybody experiences fat being turned into muscle. If one hikes the AT to lose weight, the real challenge regarding body weight is keeping the lost weight from coming back after the hike.

Equipment List for Appalachian Trail Hike in 2016 and 2017	Start Hike	First Rev.	Sec. Rev.	Day Hike
Backpack				
ULA 75 Liter Catalyst Pack	48.00 oz.			
Pack Liner Bag / air tap valve	1.80 oz.	1.80 oz.	1.80 oz.	
Stuff sack for Air Mattress			1.25 oz.	
Z-Packs Arc Blast		22.00 oz.		
Peregrine 25 Liter Day Pack			5.85 oz.	5.85 oz.
DIY hip belt with belt pockets			5.40 oz.	
Day Pack & hip belt replaced / pack below				
Z-Packs 38 Liter Nero / Belt Pockets				
Backpack Total Weight	49.80 oz.	23.80 oz.	14.30 oz.	5.85 oz.
	3.11 lbs.	1.49 lbs.	0.89 lbs.	0.37 lbs.
Shelter System				
Z-packs Duplex tent with stakes	26.50 oz.	26.50 oz.		
DIY tarp and bathtub floor / stakes			16.50 oz.	
Shelter Total Weight	26.50 oz.	26.50 oz.	16.50 oz.	0.00 oz.
	1.66 lbs.	1.66 lbs.	1.03 lbs.	0.00 lbs.
Sleep System				
Neo-Air Air mattress	17.75 oz.	17.75 oz.	17.75 oz.	
Sleeping bag liner around mattress	3.00 oz.	3.00 oz.		
DIY top-sheet for Neo-Air			2.00 oz.	
Marmott Mummy Sleeping Bag	44.90 oz.			
Go-Lite 30º Quilt		21.00 oz.	21.00 oz.	
Big Sky International Air Pillow	3.60 oz.	3.60 oz.		
Frogg Toggs stuff sack & Pillow Cover	1.20 oz.	1.20 oz.	1.20 oz.	
Z-Packs Down Hood	1.30 oz.		1.30 oz.	
Sleep System (Total Weight)	71.75 oz.	46.55 oz.	43.25 oz.	0.00 oz.
	4.48 lbs.	2.91 lbs.	2.70 lbs.	0.00 lbs.
Rain Gear				
Marmot Precept Jacket	13.90 oz.			
Berkhause Jacket		3.65 oz.	3.65 oz.	3.65 oz.
DIY Rain Kilt	1.50 oz.	1.50 oz.	1.50 oz.	1.50 oz.
DIY Pack Cover	1.50 oz.			
Rain Gear Total Weight	16.90 oz.	5.15 oz.	5.15 oz.	5.15 oz.
	1.06 lbs.	0.32 lbs.	0.32 lbs.	0.32 lbs.
Hydration System				
Sawyer Mini Squeeze	2.00 oz.			
Sawyer Regular Squeeze Filter		3.00 oz.		
Katadyn BE Free Water filter / bottle			2.55 oz.	2.55 oz.
Sawyer Squeeze Bag	1.00 oz.	1.00 oz.		
2 liter Platypus Squeeze Bottle	1.00 oz.			
1 Liter Smart Water Bottle	1.00 oz.			
28 oz. Smart Water Bottle (qty 2)	2.00 oz.	2.00 oz.	2.00 oz.	2.00 oz.
DIY Drinking Tube with Bite Valve	1.25 oz.	1.25 oz.	1.25 oz.	1.25 oz.
DIY Plastic Dipping Cup	0.20 oz.	0.20 oz.		
Hydration System Total Weight	8.45 oz.	7.45 oz.	5.80 oz.	5.80 oz.
	0.53 lbs.	0.47 lbs.	0.36 lbs.	0.36 lbs.

Equipment List for Appalachian Trail Hike in 2016 and 2017   *Page 2*

	Start Hike	First Rev.	Sec. Rev.	Day Hike
Clothing Carried *(*Carried or worn)*				
Lightweight T Shirt*	4.20oz.	4.20oz.		
OR Lightweight T Shirt*			3.45 oz.	
Quick Dry Hiking Shorts*	3.40oz.	3.40oz.	3.40 oz.	
Darn Tuff Sox	2.70oz.	2.70oz.	2.70 oz.	2.70oz.
Bug Head Net	0.60oz.	0.60oz.	0.60 oz.	0.60oz.
Buff	1.45oz.	oz.	1.45 oz.	oz.
Clothing Carried Total Weight	23.85oz.	12.35oz.	11.60 oz.	3.30oz.
	1.49lbs.	0.77lbs.	0.73lbs.	0.21lbs.
Misc. Items				
Hand Sanitizer	1.70oz.	1.70oz.	1.70 oz.	1.00oz.
Selfie Holder	0.80oz.			
Bear Bag System	4.30oz.	4.30oz.		
Bear Bag Chest Pack with rope			3.25 oz.	
Pee Bottle	1.90oz.	1.90oz.	1.90 oz.	
Pepper Spray	3.00oz.			
Camp Slippers (foam)	2.20oz.			
Garmin inReach Explorer				7.50oz.
Dual Phone Charger / cord	4.30oz.	4.30oz.	4.30 oz.	
Phone Recharger Battery / cord	6.25oz.	6.25oz.	6.25 oz.	4.00oz.
Misc. Items Total Weight	24.45oz.	18.45oz.	17.40 oz.	12.50oz.
	1.53lbs.	1.15lbs.	1.09 lbs.	0.78lbs.
Cooking System *(Individual wt. not shown)*				
750 mm Titanium Cook pot / lid	X	X	X	
Titanium Wind Screen	X	X	X	
DIY Fancy Feast Alcohol Stove	X	X		
DIY Refletex Cozy / stuff sack	X	X	X	
MSR Folding long handled spoon	X	X	X	
Bic Mini Lighter	X	X	X	
Esbit Stove			X	
Hand soap leaves		X	X	X
Small Swiss Army Knife	X			
Derma-Safe Folding Utility Razor		X	X	X
Cooking System Total Weight	9.25oz.	7.00oz.	7.00 oz.	0.40oz.
	0.58lbs.	0.44lbs.	0.44 lbs.	0.03lbs.

* These items are either worn or are carried, depending upon the weather. Their weight is only added in once.

Equipment List for Appalachian Trail Hike in 2016 and 2017 Page 3				
	Start Hike	First Rev.	Sec. Rev.	Day Hike
Ditty Bag / Personal Hygiene, First Aid, & Elect. Items (Individual wts not shown)				
Sleeping Pills	X	X	X	X
Imodium AD	X	X	X	X
Benadryl Pills	X	X	X	X
Ibuprofen	X	X	X	X
Prescribed Med for Tendonitis	X	X	X	
Antibiotic for Lyme Disease	X	X	X	
Steroid Liquid for Poison Ivy	X	X	X	
100% Deet	X	X	X	X
K T Tape			X	X
Second Skin	X	X	X	X
Band-Aids	X	X	X	X
Antiseptic Wipes	X	X	X	X
3 in 1 Antibiotic	X	X	X	X
Bee Sting Wipes	X	X	X	X
Tooth Brush and Tooth Paste	X	X	X	
Bic Mini Lighter (backup)	X			
Paper Book Matches		X	X	X
Fire Starter	X	X	X	X
Mini Compass	X	X	X	X
Tweezers		X	X	X
Compressed Paper Hand towel	X	X	X	X
Air Mattress Repair Patches	X	X	X	
Tick Removal Key	X	X	X	
Needle / Dental Floss for Repairs	X	X	X	X
Safety Pins	X	X	X	X
Duct Tape	X	X	X	X
Leukotape P Sports Tape			X	X
Rip stop Repair Tape	X	X	X	X
Cuban Fiber Repair Tape	X	X	X	X
Dr. Bonner's Liquid Soap	X	X		
Soap Leaves			X	X
Lip Balm	X	X	X	X
Writing paper and pen	X	X	X	X
Lightweight 1/16" cord 10 ft.	X	X	X	X
Toilet Paper	X	X	X	X
Salt/Pepper	X	X		
Katadyn Purification tablets	X	X	X	X
Black Diamond Head Lamp	X	X	X	X
AAA Batteries for Headlamp (2)	X	X		
Small Thumb Sized Flashlight	X	X	X	X
Backup Batteries for Flashlight	X	X	X	X
Ear Phones	X	X	X	X
Plastic container to hold stuff	X			
Plastic bag to hold stuff		X	X	X
Ditty Bag Total Weight	16.00 oz.	10.00 oz.	7.40 oz.	4.20 oz.
	1.00 lbs.	0.63 lbs.	0.46 lbs.	0.26 lbs.

Equipment List for Appalachian Trail Hike in 2016 and 2017			Page 4
	Start Hike	First Rev.	Sec. Rev.	Day Hike
Items Worn or Carried on Body				
Exofficial Hiking Shirt*	8.10 oz.	8.10 oz.	8.10 oz.	
Lightweight T Shirt*				
OR Lightweight T Shirt*				3.45 oz.
Exofficial Convertible Pants with Belt*	8.10 oz.	8.10 oz.	8.10 oz.	
Exofficial Convertible Pants Legs*	3.75 oz.			
Quick Dry Hiking Shorts*				3.40 oz.
Darn Tuff Sox	2.70 oz.	2.70 oz.	2.70 oz.	2.70 oz.
Under Armour Underwear	3.00 oz.	3.00 oz.	3.00 oz.	
Exofficial Underware				1.60 oz.
HeadSweats Ball Cap	2.00 oz.	2.00 oz.	2.00 oz.	2.00 oz.
DIY Neck Shade from Cooling Towel	1.20 oz.	1.20 oz.	1.20 oz.	1.20 oz.
Dirty Girl Gators	1.30 oz.	1.30 oz.		
Solomon Hiking Shoes w/ Sole insoles	39.00 oz.			
HOKA Trail Runner Shoes / Insoles		32.60 oz.	32.60 oz.	32.60 oz.
Watch, Casio SGW-300H			1.65 oz.	1.65 oz.
Eye Glasses with Neck Holder	2.50 oz.	2.50 oz.	2.50 oz.	2.50 oz.
Fizan Trekking Poles	18.00 oz.	18.00 oz.		
PacerPoles			19.30 oz.	19.30 oz.
DIY Cuban billfold	2.00 oz.	2.00 oz.	2.00 oz.	2.00 oz.
Droid Turbo 2 Cell Phone (Verizon)	6.00 oz.	6.00 oz.	6.00 oz.	
Droid Z Turbo / extra battery				9.15 oz.
Weight of Items Worn or Carried	97.65 oz.	87.50 oz.	89.15 oz.	81.55 oz.
	6.10 lbs.	5.47 lbs.	5.57 lbs.	5.10 lbs.
Consumables for four days (except day hiking)				
Toilet Paper	6.00 oz.	2.00 oz.	2.00 oz.	2.00 oz.
Fuel	12.00 oz.	4.00 oz.	4.00 oz.	0.00 oz.
Water	64.00 oz.	64.00 oz.	42.00 oz.	42.00 oz.
Food (8 oz. a meal)	80.00 oz.	80.00 oz.	80.00 oz.	12.00 oz.
Food (Safety Margin)	80.00 oz.	20.00 oz.	10.00 oz.	0.00 oz.
Consumables Total Weight	242.00 oz.	170.00 oz.	138.00 oz.	56.00 oz.
	15.13 lbs.	10.63 lbs.	8.63 lbs.	3.50 lbs.
Total Pack Base Weight	246.95 oz.	157.25 oz.	128.40 oz.	37.20 oz.
	15.43 lbs.	9.83 lbs.	8.03 lbs.	2.33 lbs.
Total Pack Weight with Consumables	488.95 oz.	327.25 oz.	266.40 oz.	93.20 oz.
	30.56 lbs.	20.45 lbs.	16.65 lbs.	5.83 lbs.
Total Items Worn or Carried on Body	97.65 oz.	87.50 oz.	89.15 oz.	81.55 oz.
	6.10 lbs.	5.47 lbs.	5.57 lbs.	5.10 lbs.
Total Skin Out Weight	586.60 oz.	414.75 oz.	355.55 oz.	174.75 oz.
	36.66 lbs.	25.92 lbs.	22.22 lbs.	10.92 lbs.

* These items are worn or are carried, depending upon the weather. Weight is only added in once.

How to "Hire a Sherpa" for 50 Cents a Mile to Carry Half of Your Base Weight!

Earlier, I explained how I was hiking from Springer Mountain, hikers just starting their hike were everywhere. Because I had already hiked 900 miles and had learned the importance of carrying a small pack, others were naturally interested in what was in my pack as well as what was not in it. After explaining their pack size was in direct proportion to their fears, the concept of lightweight equipment still seemed to elude a majority. To help this group overcome this mental block, I started telling people they should hire a Sherpa who would carry half their pack base weight for only 50 cents a mile! I told them the Sherpa wanted all his money up front, but he would take it on a credit card. Naturally, this all raised a lot of curiosity. I then would explain how to hire a Sherpa for 50 cents a mile.

I said, "Take a thousand dollars and replace your equipment with lightweight equipment then send home the replaced items as well as the items you will not need, and you have effectively hired a Sherpa to carry half your base weight. OR, get a box and instead of sending stuff home, send it to yourself on up the trail a few days. When you catch up with your box, either send it home or keep sending it up the trail until you realize you simply don't need all the items you originally thought you would need."

Because of this conversation, as well as encouraging hikers to day hike and avoid carrying a full backpack, I gave myself the challenge to create a full pack with a base weight of fewer than 10 pounds and at the cost of less than a thousand dollars. Why tie up a lot of money if you are only going to use the equipment for a few nights on the trail? This list is the results of that challenge.

Please note I included a few upgrade items at the end of the list that will raise the cost but also lower the weight. If I were going to do any upgrading, I would start with the sleeping quilt, then the upgraded tent, and finally the pack. The upgraded quilt saves half a pound but also gives one a great piece of equipment to be used when car camping as well as at some hostels. If car camping and sleeping in a tent most nights, this upgrade would be well worth the extra $20.00 and 3 ounces. In fact, if I did not need ever to carry the tent I was using to car camp, I'd probably get one that I could stand up in as well as set up in a very short time. Because weight would not even be an issue, the tent would be very roomie along with an extremely comfortable air mattress or even a cot. I would probably also go with a propane gas stove with a griddle. One might as well as have the car camping gear based on comfort and ease of use instead of weight.

"Hire a Sherpa" to carry half your base weight for less than 50 cents a mile!

	Ounces	Price	Ounces	Price
Backpack				
G4Free Large 40L Lightweight Backpack	11.70oz.	$18.99		
Pack Liner Bag	1.00oz.	$1.00		
Backpack Total Weight and Price			12.70.oz.	$19.99
Shelter System				
Six Moons Design Lunar Solo Tent	24.00oz.	$225.00		
MSR GroundHog Stake Kit	3.00oz.	$14.35		
Shelter Total Weight and Price			27.00.oz.	$239.35
Sleep System				
AEGISMAX Ultra-Light 95% Down Sleeping Bag	24.60oz.	$107.00		
Outdoorsman Lab Ultralight Sleeping Pad	14.50oz.	$39.97		
Klymit Pillow X Inflatable Pillow	1.95	$16.23		
Sleep System Total Weight and Price			41.05.oz.	$163.20
Rain Gear				
Fogg Toggs Ultra-Lite Men's Rain Suit	10.20oz.	$24.99		
Rain Gear Total Weight and Price			10.20.oz.	$24.99
Hydration System				
Katadyn BE Free Water filter with bottle	2.55oz.	$35.00		
28 oz. Smart Water Bottle (quantity 2)	2.00oz.	$3.00		
DIY Drinking Tube with Bite Valve	1.25oz.	$15.00		
Hydration System Total Weight and Price			5.80.oz.	$53.00
Clothing Carried (*Carried or worn, depending on weather*)				
*Lightweight T Shirt	6.00oz.	$10.00		
*Quick Dry Hiking Shorts	6.00oz.	$10.00		
Darn Tuff Sox	2.70oz.	$20.00		
Lightweight Underware of Choice	4.00oz.	$15.00		
4YANG Packable Lightweight Spring Down Jacket	10.00oz.	$15.00		
Buff for Head and Neck (and pillow covering)	1.40oz.	$10.00		
Plastic zip lock gallon bag (2) to hold clothing	1.00	$0.50		
*Bug Head Net (also stuff sack for cooking kit)	0.60oz.	$5.00		
Clothing Carried Total Weight and Price		$85.50	31.70.oz.	$85.50
Misc. Items				
Hand Sanitizer	1.70oz.	$1.50		
Bear Bag System	4.30oz.	$30.00		
Black Diamond Ion Headlamp	1.90oz.	$24.95		
AAA Batteries for Headlamp (2)	1.50oz.	$2.00		
Cell Phone Recharger Battery with cord	5.50oz.	$30.00		
Misc. Items Total Weight and Price			14.90.oz.	$88.45

"Hire a Sherpa" to carry half your base weight for less than 50 cents a mile! **Page 2**

	Ounces	Price	Ounces	Price
Cooking System *(Individual weights & prices not shown)*				
750 mm Titanium Cook pot with lid		x		
Aluminum Foil Wind Screen		x		
DIY Fancy Feast Alcohol Stove		x		
DIY Refletex Cozy and stuff sack		x		
Plastic spoon		x		
Mini Bic Lighter		x		
Plastic bottle for alcohol		x		
Small Knife		x		
Cooking System Total Weight and Price			7.50.oz.	$65.00

Plastic Ditty Bag with Hygiene, First Aid, and Elect. Items *(Individual weights & prices not shown)*

	Ounces	Price	Ounces	Price
Imodium AD Pills		X		
Benadryl Pills		X		
Ibuprofen Pills		X		
100% Deet Insect Repellant		X		
Mole Skin		X		
K T Tape		X		
Band-Aids		X		
Antiseptic Wipes		X		
3 in 1 Antibiotic		X		
Benadryl Cream		X		
Tooth Brush and Tooth Paste		X		
Paper Book Matches		X		
Mini Compass		X		
Tweezers		X		
Air Mattress Repair Patches		X		
Needle with Dental Floss for Sewing Repairs		X		
Safety Pins		X		
Duct Tape		X		
Clear Repair Tape for Air Mattress Repair		X		
Soap Sheets		X		
Lightweight 1/16" cord 10 ft.		X		
Katadyn Purification tablets		X		
Small Thumb Sized Flashlight		X		
Backup Batteries for Thumb Sized Flashlight		X		
Ear Phones		X		
Ditty Bag Total Weight and Price			5.50.oz.	$60.00

Total Base Weight	156.35.oz.
	9.77 lbs.

Total Price of Equipment Carried before shipping and taxes	$799.48

"Hire a Sherpa" to carry half your base weight for less than 50 cents a mile! **Page 3**

	Ounces	Price	Ounces	Price
Higher end substitutions	Plus (minus)			
Zpacks Nero Backpack	(0.80) oz.	$180.00		
Enlightened Equipment Enigma 30° Quilt	(8.60) oz.	$173.00		
Six Moons Design Skyscape Trekker Tent	3.00 oz.	$20.00		
Complementary clothing/equipment to be worn or carried on person				
Lightweight Long "roll-up" Sleeve Fishing Shirt	8.00 oz.	$22.00		
Convertible Long Pants with zip off Legs	13.00 oz.	$25.00		
Darn Tough Sox	2.70 oz.	$20.00		
Lightweight Underware of Choice	4.00 oz.	$15.00		
Hat of choice	3.00 oz.	$10.00		
New Balance 481V3 Cushioning Trail Running Shoe	16.00 oz.	$50.00		
Cell Phone of choice (cost not figured in pricing)	6.00 oz.	0.00		
Cascade Mountain Tech Carbon Trekking Poles	15.00 oz.	$44.00		
	67.70 oz.	$186.00		
	4.23 lbs.			
Total Equipment Weight			14.00 lbs.	
Total Price before shipping and taxes				$985.48
Complementary items as needed				
Poly Lightweight Top & Bottom / Underwear Guys	10.00 oz.	$26.00		

Nutrition Charts

These charts are provided to assist in the planning of food for long-distance hiking. They include both trail food and town food. The first chart has foods sorted in alphabetical order. The second chart has food sorted by calorie by the ounce to show calorie density. The final chart shows the nutritional value of town food, energy foods, and energy drinks.

The first column lists the food item. The second column lists the calories per ounce or calories per serving for town food. The third, fourth, and fifth columns show grams per ounce of fats, carbohydrates, and proteins. I found the best mix that gave me the most energy was to eat a ratio of 3 grams of carbohydrates to 2 grams of fats to 1 gram of protein.

Food Sorted by Calorie Density

Food (Typical for similar items)	Calories per Ounce	Fat grams per Ounce	Carb grams per Ounce	Protein grams per Ounce
Oil, Olive	240	28	0	0
Butter, Hazelnut	182	17	5	4
Butter, Cashew	174	15	9	4
Peanuts	170	15	4	8
Nuts, Almond	167	15	6	6
Butter, Peanut	166	14	6	7
Corn Chips, Frito®	160	10	15	2
Potato Chips, Lay's® Plain	160	10	15	2
Butter, Justin's® Chocolate Hazelnut	159	12	11	4
Nuts, Cashew	157	13	3	5
Nutella®	154	8	17	2
Doritos®	150	8	17	2
Cheese and Crackers, Lance Captain's®	145	7	17	2
Bar, Kind®	143	11	11	4
Crackers, White Cheez-It®	140	7	17	3
Hueos Rancheros, Backpacker's Pantry	140	7	7	11
Pepperoni, Sliced	140	13	0	5
Granola	139	7	15	4
Cracker, Pepperidge Farm Original Goldfish	136	5	18	3
Bar, Snickers®	135	6	18	2
Mix, Sweet 'n Salty Trail	135	9	14	4
Bar, Clif® Chocolate Chip Builder's Protein	133	1	13	8
Cookies, Oreo®	133	6	21	1
Mix, Trail	131	8	13	4
Crackers, BelVita® Breakfast	131	5	20	2
Bar, Granola	128	5	19	2
Noodles, Ramen	127	5	17	3
Bar, Gatorade® Whey Protein	125	4	15	7
Buns, Little Debbie® Honey	125	7	15	2
Honey Buns, Little Debbie's	125	7	15	2
Soybeans, Edamame® Freeze Dried Green	124	6	9	11
Lasagna, Alpineaire Three Cheese	122	2	21	6
Chex Mix®	120	4	22	2
Corn, Simply Balanced® Freeze Dried Sweet	120	3	20	4
Rice and Chicken, Mountain House®	120	4	18	3
Pork, Mountain House Sweet and Sour	119	2	20	5
Apples, Freeze Dried	117	0	27	2
Bar, Trail Mix Bar Granola	117	3	21	3
Beans, Santa Fe Instant SW Style Refried	116	2	17	6
Bar, Rice Krispies® Treat	115	3	22	1
Pan Thai, Good To-Go®	115	3	19	4
Cheese, Cheddar	114	9	0	7
Cheese, Hard	114	9	0	7
Pasta, Knorr® Sides	114	2	20	4
Bar, Backpacker Pucks	113	5	16	3

Food Sorted by Calorie Density   Page 2

Food (Typical for similar items)	Calories per Ounce	Fat grams per Ounce	Carb grams per Ounce	Protein grams per Ounce
Cereal, Cheerios Honey Nut® Dry	111	2	22	2
Donut, Glazed	110	6	12	1
Sticks, Cooked Salami	110	9	2	5
Stuffing, Stove Top	110	1	21	4
Sugar, White	110	0	28	0
Soup, Lipton Dry Chicken Noodle Cup-of-	109	2	17	4
Pop-tart®	109	3	21	1
Couscous	107	0	22	4
Posta, Kraft® Mac and Cheese	107	2	20	3
Oatmeal, Instant	107	1	21	3
Rice, Knorr® Sides (Various)	105	1	21	3
Fruit Leathers	105	1	24	0
Roll, Cinnamon Sweet with Raisons	105	5	14	2
Bar, Clif®	104	2	19	4
Soup, Dry Creamy Asparagus	104	3	16	4
Potatoes, Mashed	102	0	22	3
Breakfast, Carnation Instant (Various)	102	0	21	4
Cookies, Nabisco® Fig Newtons	101	2	20	1
Leather, Fruit	101	2	24	0
Cherries, Dried	100	1	24	2
Peach's, Freeze Dried	100	0	27	0
Strawberry's, Freeze Dried	100	0	24	2
Cheese, Cream	99	10	1	2
Rice Blend, Quick Cook	99	1	19	3
Banana, Dried	98	1	25	1
Chile, Good To-Go® Smoked Three Bean	97	1	18	5
Lentils	95	0	17	7
Cranberries, Ocean Spray® Craisin's® Dried	92	0	23	0
Pineapple, Dried	92	1	22	1
Bar, Special K (Kellogg's) Blueberry	90	2	18	1
Pie, Fried Fruit	90	5	12	1
Honey	86	0	23	0
Raisins	85	0	22	1
Tortilla, Flour	85	2	15	2
Spam® Singles Classic	83	7	1	4
Bagel, Whole Wheat	80	1	15	3
Jerky, Jack Link's® Beef	80	1	3	15
Bagel, Plain	78	1	15	3
Bread, Whole Wheat	73	1	13	3
Jelly (average), Smucker's®	71	0	18	0
Bread, Albertson's Flat	69	2	11	2
Apricots, Dried	68	0	18	1
Salmon Foil Packet, Pink	28	1	0	5
Tuna Foil Packet, Ranch Flavor	27	0	0	6
Milk, Non-Fat Dry	25	0	4	3

Town Food Sorted by Calorie Density Page 3

Town Food (Typical for similar items)	Calories per Ounce	Fat grams per Ounce	Carb grams per Ounce	Protein grams per Ounce
McDonalds Big Breakfast with Pancakes	1350	65	155	35
Olive Garden Dinner Fettuccine Alfredo	1219	75	99	36
Olive Garden Dinner Spaghetti with Meat Sauce	709	22	94	36
Duncan Donuts Croissant Sausage, Egg, and Cheese	700	50	41	23
Duncan Donuts Bagel Sausage, Egg, and Cheese	680	33	67	28
Duncan Donuts Ciabatta Chicken, Bacon, Cheese	580	22	63	32
McDonalds Big Mac	540	28	46	25
KFC Extra Crispy Chicken Breast	530	35	18	35
Subway 6" Flat Bread Bacon, Egg, and Cheese	460	21	43	25
McDonalds Bacon, Egg & Cheese Biscuit	450	24	40	18
McDonalds Double Cheese Burger	430	21	35	25
Subway 6" Sweet Onion Chicken Teriyaki	370	4	25	25
McDonalds McChicken	350	15	40	15
McDonalds Medium Fries	340	16	44	4
Papa Johns 12" Medium, Pan Dough Crust, Pepperoni	330	14	35	15
KFC Original Chicken Breast, with Skin & Breading	320	19	9	33
Subway 6" Club	310	5	46	23
Duncan Donuts Glazed Croissant Donut	310	16	36	5
McDonalds 6 Piece Chicken McNuggets	270	16	16	15
Papa Johns 12" Medium, Original Crust, Pepperoni	260	12	27	13
McDonalds Apple Pie	240	10	33	2
KFC Grilled Chicken Breast	180	6	0	31
McDonalds Hash browns	150	9	16	1
Olive Garden Bread Stick with Garlic Butter	140	2	26	5

Energy Food (May contain sodium, caffeine, Potassium, & Amino Acids)				
Beans, Jelly Belly Assorted flavors	100	0	25	0
Gu Energy Gel	100	2	21	0
Gatorade Chews	95	0	23	0

Drinks (May contain sodium, caffeine, Potassium, & Amino Acids)				
Fruit Smoothie Naked Mighty Mango	290	0	68	2
Gatorade Perform Thirst Quencher Drink Power	60	0	14	0
Mix, Crystal Light with Caffeine Strawberry	10	0	0	0
Mix, Great Value Peach Mango Energy Drink	10	0	0	0

Food Sorted by Name

Food (Typical for similar items)	Calories per Ounce	Fat grams per Ounce	Carb grams per Ounce	Protein grams per Ounce
Apples, Freeze Dried	117	0	27	2
Apricots, Dried	68	0	18	1
Bagel, Plain	78	1	15	3
Bagel, Whole Wheat	80	1	15	3
Banana, Dried	98	1	25	1
Bar, Backpacker Pucks	113	5	16	3
Bar, Clif®	104	2	19	4
Bar, Clif® Chocolate Chip Builder's Protein	133	1	13	8
Bar, Gatorade® Whey Protein	125	4	15	7
Bar, Granola	128	5	19	2
Bar, Kind®	143	11	11	4
Bar, Rice Krispies® Treat	115	3	22	1
Bar, Snickers®	135	6	18	2
Bar, Special K (Kellogg's) Blueberry	90	2	18	1
Bar, Trail Mix Bar Granola	117	3	21	3
Beans, Santa Fe Instant SW Style Refried	116	2	17	6
Bread, Albertson's Flat	69	2	11	2
Bread, Whole Wheat	73	1	13	3
Breakfast, Carnation Instant (Various)	102	0	21	4
Buns, Little Debbie® Honey	125	7	15	2
Butter, Cashew	174	15	9	4
Butter, Hazelnut	182	17	5	4
Butter, Justin's® Chocolate Hazelnut	159	12	11	4
Butter, Peanut	166	14	6	7
Cereal, Cheerios Honey Nut® Dry	111	2	22	2
Cheese and Crackers, Lance Captain's®	145	7	17	2
Cheese, Cheddar	114	9	0	7
Cheese, Cream	99	10	1	2
Cheese, Hard	114	9	0	7
Cherries, Dried	100	1	24	2
Chex Mix®	120	4	22	2
Chile, Good To-Go® Smoked Three Bean	97	1	18	5
Cookies, Nabisco® Fig Newtons	101	2	20	1
Cookies, Oreo®	133	6	21	1
Corn Chips, Frito®	160	10	15	2
Corn, Simply Balanced® Freeze Dried Sweet	120	3	20	4
Couscous	107	0	22	4
Cracker, Pepperidge Farm Original Goldfish	136	5	18	3
Crackers, BelVita® Breakfast	131	5	20	2
Crackers, White Cheez-It®	140	7	17	3
Cranberries, Ocean Spray® Craisin's® Dried	92	0	23	0
Donut, Glazed	110	6	12	1
Doritos®	150	8	17	2
Fruit Leathers	105	1	24	0
Granola	139	7	15	4

Food Sorted by Name Page 2

Food (Typical for similar items)	Calories per Ounce	Fat grams per Ounce	Carb grams per Ounce	Protein grams per Ounce
Honey	86	0	23	0
Honey Buns, Little Debbie's	125	7	15	2
Hueos Rancheros, Backpacker's Pantry	140	7	7	11
Jelly (average), Smucker's®	71	0	18	0
Jerky, Jack Link's® Beef	80	1	3	15
Lasagna, Alpineaire Three Cheese	122	2	21	6
Leather, Fruit	101	2	24	0
Lentils	95	0	17	7
Milk, Non-Fat Dry	25	0	4	3
Mix, Sweet 'n Salty Trail	135	9	14	4
Mix, Trail	131	8	13	4
Noodles, Ramen	127	5	17	3
Nutella®	154	8	17	2
Nuts, Almond	167	15	6	6
Nuts, Cashew	157	13	3	5
Oatmeal, Instant	107	1	21	3
Oil, Olive	240	28	0	0
Pan Thai, Good To-Go®	115	3	19	4
Pasta, Knorr® Sides	114	2	20	4
Peach's, Freeze Dried	100	0	27	0
Peanuts	170	15	4	8
Pepperoni, Sliced	140	13	0	5
Pie, Fried Fruit	90	5	12	1
Pineapple, Dried	92	1	22	1
Pop-tart®	109	3	21	1
Pork, Mountain House Sweet and Sour	119	2	20	5
Posta, Kraft® Mac and Cheese	107	2	20	3
Potato Chips, Lay's® Plain	160	10	15	2
Potatoes, Mashed	102	0	22	3
Raisins	85	0	22	1
Rice and Chicken, Mountain House®	120	4	18	3
Rice Blend, Quick Cook	99	1	19	3
Rice, Knorr® Sides (Various)	105	1	21	3
Roll, Cinnamon Sweet with Raisons	105	5	14	2
Salmon Foil Packet, Pink	28	1	0	5
Soup, Dry Creamy Asparagus	104	3	16	4
Soup, Lipton Dry Chicken Noodle Cup-of-	109	2	17	4
Soybeans, Edamame® Freeze Dried Green	124	6	9	11
Spam® Singles Classic	83	7	1	4
Sticks, Cooked Salami	110	9	2	5
Strawberry's, Freeze Dried	100	0	24	2
Stuffing, Stove Top	110	1	21	4
Sugar, White	110	0	28	0
Tortilla, Flour	85	2	15	2
Tuna Foil Packet, Ranch Flavor	27	0	0	6

Town Food Sorted by Calorie Density   Page 3

Town Food (Typical for similar items)	Calories per Ounce	Fat grams per Ounce	Carb grams per Ounce	Protein grams per Ounce
Duncan Donuts Bagel Sausage, Egg, and Cheese	680	33	67	28
Duncan Donuts Ciabatta Chicken, Bacon, Cheese	580	22	63	32
Duncan Donuts Croissant Sausage, Egg, and Cheese	700	50	41	23
Duncan Donuts Glazed Croissant Donut	310	16	36	5
KFC Extra Crispy Chicken Breast	530	35	18	35
KFC Grilled Chicken Breast	180	6	0	31
KFC Original Chicken Breast, with Skin & Breading	320	19	9	33
McDonalds 6 Piece Chicken McNuggets	270	16	16	15
McDonalds Apple Pie	240	10	33	2
McDonalds Bacon, Egg & Cheese Biscuit	450	24	40	18
McDonalds Big Breakfast with Pancakes	1350	65	155	35
McDonalds Big Mac	540	28	46	25
McDonalds Double Cheese Burger	430	21	35	25
McDonalds Hash browns	150	9	16	1
McDonalds McChicken	350	15	40	15
McDonalds Medium Fires	340	16	44	4
Olive Garden Bread Stick with Garlic Butter	140	2	26	5
Olive Garden Dinner Fettuccine Alfredo	1219	75	99	36
Olive Garden Dinner Spaghetti with Meat Sauce	709	22	94	36
Papa Johns 12" Medium, Original Crust, Pepperoni	260	12	27	13
Papa Johns 12" Medium, Pan Dough Crust, Pepperoni	330	14	35	15
Subway 6" Sweet Onion Chicken Teriyaki	370	4	25	25
Subway 6" Club	310	5	46	23
Subway 6" Flat Bread Bacon, Egg, and Cheese	460	21	43	25

Energy Food (May contain sodium, caffeine, Potassium, & Amino Acids)

Beans, Jelly Belly Assorted flavors	100	0	25	0
Gatorade Chews	95	0	23	0
Gu Energy Gel	100	2	21	0

Drinks (May contain sodium, caffeine, Potassium, & Amino Acids)

Fruit Smoothie Naked Mighty Mango	290	0	68	2
Gatorade Perform Thirst Quencher Drink Power	60	0	14	0
Mix, Crystal Light with Caffeine Strawberry	10	0	0	0
Mix, Great Value Peach Mango Energy Drink	10	0	0	0

Terms or Definitions

Aqua Blazing

Floating down a river instead of hiking the trail and following the white blazes.

AT

Appalachian Trail

ATC

Appalachian Trail Conservatory or ATC is the organization tasked with managing the entire Appalachian Trail. They are headquartered in Harpers Ferry. They have an extensive library of information on their website, www.appalachiantrail.org.

Awol or Awol's Guide

An Appalachian Trail guidebook titled *The A.T. Guide* and published by former thru-hiker, David Miller, with the trail name of Awol. This guidebook is one of two major guidebooks giving similar trail information. The other book is called *Thru-Hikers' Companion* which is published by the Appalachian Trail Conservatory or ATC.

Balds

Mountain or hilltops that have no trees but are covered with open grasslands or rocky ledges.

Base weight

The weight of a pack when loaded with all the equipment to be carried. Does not include consumables such as water, food, fuel, toilet paper and Ibuprofen

Blazes

Marks that show the location of a trail. The AT is marked with 2 inch by 6 inch white blazes.

Blue Blazes

Blue paint marks trails that lead to features along the AT such as campsites, springs, privies, parking lots, great sights and a variety of other places. Also marks trails that are alternatives to be taken, such as severe weather trails that avoid an exposed ridge that would be unsafe to hike during severe weather.

Bobo

Both Bound meaning a hiker that is hiking the AT by hiking some of the times north and some of the time south. Also called Flip-Flop hiking.

Bubble

A large group of hikers, generally referred to as the hiker bubble that starts at Springer Mountain in the spring and heads north.

Cameling Up

Drinking a large amount of water, generally at a water source.

CDT

Continental Divide Trail, one of the three major hiking trails in the United States. It runs from Mexico to Canada along the United States continental divide.

Cozy

An insulated covering used to help retain heat from adding hot water to dehydrated food. Speeds up cooking time.

Day Hiking

Hiking just for one day, not carrying equipment or gear to stay overnight on the trail. Also called "Slack Packing."

DIY

Do It Yourself refers to making your gear or doing something yourself.

Elbow Bump

Bumping elbows instead of shaking hands. Helps stop the spread of diseases such as Norovirus. Fist bumps are also used in this same way.

Esbit

Trade name for a solid stove fuel that comes in a small brick or pill form.

Fist Bump

Bumping fists instead of shaking hands. Helps stop the spread of diseases such as Norovirus. Elbow bumps are also used in this way.

FKT

Fastest Known Time. Used as a method of tracking speed records on trails.

Flip-Flop

Hiking in one direction then changing to hiking in the opposite direction. Often used by northbound thru-hikers who are running out of time to reach Katahdin before it closes in the fall. By jumping up to Katahdin and hiking south, this problem is alleviated. Another example of a Flip-Flop hike is starting in the middle of the trail, hiking to the end and then returning to the starting point and hiking in the opposite direction to the other end of the trail.

Sometimes called a BoBo meaning "both directions."

Guthook

A smartphone app that is a GPS, guidebook, map, and general information provider to hikers on all major trails. Most thru-hikers see this app as a must-have.

Hiker Hunger

After a person has been hiking a few days or weeks, the body will start begging for more food. This is called hiker hunger. This also will cause hikers to gain weight after a long-distance hike.

Hiker Midnight

The time in the evening, after dinner, when hikers start to get ready for bed. Generally, around sundown.

Hostel

A shared-room or dormitory-like accommodation that caters to individual travelers. Most have a variety of services needed by backpackers and hikers.

HYOH

Hike Your Own Hike. Meaning hike in a way you want to as long as you don't impose or infringe on others.

Lightweight Backpacking

No formal definition but generally backpacking with a pack that weighs less than twenty pounds.

LNT

Leave No Trace. When you leave an area, leave the area with no evidence you had been there.

Nero

A day of hiking that is short on mileage. Not a zero (day not hiking) but near to it or a Nero.

Nobo

Northbound meaning a hiker that is hiking the AT by hiking from south to north.

PCT

Pacific Crest Trail, one of the three major hiking trails in the United States. It runs from Mexico to Canada along the Pacific mountain ranges.

PCT Bear Bag Hang

A method of hanging bear bags in trees that was developed on the Pacific Crest Trail.

Pink Blazing

Hiking in a manner to allow someone to catch a person they want to get to know better.

Privy

A bathroom designed for people to use while on the AT. Can be an elaborate building or a simple "stool" to sit on while taking a dump. Could also be called an "outhouse." Located at most shelters and some campgrounds along the AT.

Purist

A person who thinks there is only one way to hike the AT, and that is by walking by every white blaze and carrying all their gear the entire way. May have other criteria as well. Often called a Traditionalist. Could be defined as people who think everybody should hike like they hike.

REI

A major outdoor retailer named Recreational Equipment, Incorporated. They are a member-owned company.

S-Biner

An S-shaped device with dual spring gates that will hold or secure items.

Section Hiking

Hiking just a portion of the AT.

Self Double-Shuttle

A method for shuttling two to four people to and from the trail on a daily basis that uses just one vehicle and no outside shuttle driver but allows all hikers to hike in the same direction.

Shakedown

Gear shakedown is a review of what one is carrying on the trail, generally done by a person with knowledge of backpacking. A hiking shakedown is a hike that is used as a preliminary hike where a person takes all the gear they are planning on taking on a longer hike.

Shelter

A building located along the AT designed to provide overnight accommodations to hikers and backpackers. Most are three-sided, but a few are enclosed. Generally, located next to a water source, a place to pitch tents, and a privy.

Shuttle (driver)

A person who provides a taxi service along the AT, generally for pay.

Skin out weight

The weight of everything a backpacker carries, including the clothes being worn, items carried in pockets and around the neck. Also, includes not just a fully loaded pack but consumables such as water, food, fuel, toilet paper and Ibuprofen.

Slackpacking

Hiking just for one day, not carrying equipment or gear to stay overnight on the trail. Also, called Day Hiking.

Smellables

Refers to anything that has a smell that could attract animals. Examples include food, flavored drinks, sunscreen lotion, and toothpaste.

Soaking

A method of preparing food that instead of using hot water food, the food is allowed to soak in cold water for an extended time and then is eaten cold. Foods prepared this way include oatmeal, pasta, and mashed potatoes.

Sobo

South Bound meaning a hiker that is hiking the AT by hiking from north to south.

Spork

A combination spoon and fork in one eating utensil.

Traditionalist

A person who thinks there is only one way to hike the AT and that is by walking by every white blaze and carrying all their gear the entire way. May have other criteria as well. Often called a Purist.

Trail Journal

Generally, a spiral notebook found along the trail in shelters, in weatherproof boxes beside the trail, at hostels, and various other locations.

Thru-Hikers' Companion

An Appalachian Trail guidebook published by the Appalachian Trail Conservatory or ATC. This guidebook is one of two major guidebooks giving similar trail information. The other book is called *The A.T. Guide* which is published by a former thru-hiker, David Miller, with the trail name of Awol.

Trail Angel

A person who assists hikers, generally without expecting to receive compensation.

Trail Magic

Instances of help hikers receive while hiking. Trail Magic can be food, water, and other supplies either set out along the trail or can be handed out by trail angels along the trail. Can also be services provided to hikers. Trail Magic is generally provided without expectation of compensation.

Total Pack Weight

Weight of pack when loaded with all the equipment to be carried including consumables such as water, food, fuel, toilet paper and Ibuprofen

Ultralightweight Backpacking

No formal definition but generally backpacking with a pack that weighs less than 10 pounds.

Vitamin I

Trail name for the pain reliever Ibuprofen.

Yellow Blazing

Riding in a vehicle, skipping parts of the AT. Refers to the yellow stripe down the middle of a highway.

Yogi-ing

The process of trying to get people to give a hiker food without appearing to beg. Named after Yogi Bear, famous cartoon bear is known for stealing picnic baskets of food.

Zero

Taking a day off from hiking is called a Zero.

About the Author

Gail Hinshaw was born in south-central Kansas. As a son of sharecropping parents, he was fortunate to live in a community that had a Boy Scout Troop. He became a "triple crown scout," earning the God and Country Award, the rank of Eagle Scout, and was honored with Vigil Membership in the Boy Scout Honor Fraternity, The Order of the Arrow. His youth scouting career also included being a Ranger at Philmont Scout Ranch in Cimarron, New Mexico.

His professional career included being principal in his old high school at age 26, working for the Boy Scouts of America as a District Executive, and serving as a startup and turnaround professional for numerous businesses and organizations. He started several businesses of his own and ended his career as a public speaker.

His education includes two degrees in Industrial Technology as well as holding a Six Sigma Black Belt Certification in quality and process improvement. Growing up on a farm, as well as his education and work experience, gave him the knowledge, skill, and problem-solving ability to earn the trail name, Dr. Fix-it.

His hiking and backpacking experience includes hiking close to 3,000 miles with hikes in New Mexico (Philmont Scout Ranch), Colorado (various), Arizona (Grand Canyon), as well as close to 2,000 miles of the Appalachian Trail.

He is now enjoying his retirement, serving as grandad to five grandchildren, father to two outstanding children, and as husband to one very lovely lady.

Made in United States
Troutdale, OR
12/08/2023

15543775R00139